Asanas
Mudras and Bandhas
–
Awakening Ecstatic Kundalini

Yogani

From The AYP Enlightenment Series

AYP Publishing

For ordering information go to:

www.advancedyogapractices.com

Library of Congress Control Number: 2006907578

Published simultaneously in:

Nashville, Tennessee, U.S.A.
and
London, England, U.K.

This title is also available in eBook format – ISBN 0-9786496-1-3
(For Adobe Reader)

ISBN 0-9786496-0-5 (Paperback)

"You surely know that your body is a temple where the Holy Spirit lives. The Spirit is in you and is a gift from God."

Corinthians 6:19

Introduction

Like much we may encounter as we travel along our chosen spiritual path, this small volume on *Asanas, Mudras and Bandhas* presents a paradox.

In contrast to the huge, nearly exclusive emphasis on yoga asanas (postures) seen around the world today, we intentionally go lightly on them here, instead presenting a compact and efficient asana routine as preparation for sitting practices, including spinal breathing pranayama and deep meditation.

Once a balanced relationship between asanas and sitting practices is established, we move into instructions for advanced mudras and bandhas (inner physical maneuvers), which are woven into the tapestry of our daily practice routine like golden threads.

Then we cover the awakening and management of our inner ecstatic energy – *Kundalini* – and its ultimate consequences. Ecstatic awakening and its steady expansion outward through our nervous system to full divine expression is, after all, what asanas, mudras and bandhas are for.

In short, this book puts a wide range of yoga practices into perspective, moving decidedly away from the *magic bullet* single solution syndrome, and offering a clear, balanced road map for those who seek to achieve the ultimate aims of yoga. In this, asanas, mudras and bandhas have an important role to play.

The Advanced Yoga Practices Enlightenment Series is an endeavor to present the most effective methods of spiritual practice in a series of easy-to-read books that anyone can use to gain practical results immediately and over the long term. For centuries, many of these powerful practices have been shrouded in secrecy, mainly in an effort to preserve them. Now we find ourselves in the *information age*, and able to preserve knowledge for present and future generations like never before. The question remains: "How far can we go in effectively transmitting spiritual methods in writing?"

Since its beginnings in 2003, the writings of *Advanced Yoga Practices* have been an experiment to see just how much can be conveyed, with much more detail included on practices than in the spiritual writings of the past. Can books provide us the specific means necessary to tread the path to enlightenment, or do we have to surrender at the feet of a *guru* to find our salvation? Well, clearly we must surrender to something, even if it is to our own innate potential to live a freer and happier life. If we are able to do that, and maintain regular practice, then books like this one can come alive and instruct us in the ways of human spiritual transformation. If the reader is ready and the book is worthy, amazing things can happen.

While one person's name is given as the author of this book, it is actually a distillation of the efforts of thousands of practitioners over thousands of years. This is one person's attempt to simplify and make practical the spiritual methods that many have demonstrated throughout history. All who have gone before have my deepest gratitude, as do the many I am privileged to be in touch with in the present who continue to practice with dedication and good results.

I hope you will find this book to be a useful resource as you travel along your chosen path.

Practice wisely, and enjoy!

Table of Contents

Chapter 1 – The Body - Door to the Infinite

From childhood most of us are taught that we need an intermediary to find a connection to that magical *something more* in life that, down through the ages, has been referred to as *God* or *Truth*. Our priests, ministers, mullahs, gurus and rabbis promise that if we behave rightly, we will receive the everlasting rewards that have been promised. And that is *It*, the thing we vaguely conceive of as our salvation. Whatever *It* is, we often feel we are leagues away as we trip our way through the ups and downs of everyday life.

But then, once in a while, quite miraculously, we might take a long slow stretch, relax our mind, or be resting in complete stillness, and, suddenly, something vast opens up inside us – a continuum of inner peace and happiness that is as endless as it is timeless. And then, just as suddenly, we are back in the fray of life again. Where did it go, that unfathomable happiness that came from within us and then disappeared again? How can we get it back, and make it a full time experience?

When we have had such an experience (and nearly everyone has), we have been shown *the door*, so to speak. And the door is none other than us. More specifically, the door is found in the inner workings of the human nervous system. That is this nervous system, the very one we are sitting in right now. So, no matter what intermediary we have been using for guidance, in the end, it is the inner functioning of our own body that will lead us home to the *promised land*. Our body is the door to the infinite.

There is nothing new in the idea that the *kingdom of heaven* is within us. It has been around for thousands of years. But there has been so much confusion about it, you know. Throughout history, whole civilizations have risen, and fallen again, surrounded by this confusion about the true nature of humanity, first on the way up, and then on the way back down again. Will the confusion ever end?

In the meantime, over the centuries, small groups of people have been carefully collecting knowledge about the human machine – tinkering, experimenting and learning through trial and error, finding out ways to open the inner door, finding out how to open it permanently. Mostly, these people, who we tend to call saints and sages (they don't care what we call them), have labored in secret, hiding out in remote places doing their work. Once in a while a few step forward into the public eye. When the confusion gets thick enough, they do. They share their knowledge, and are often treated badly for it. It has been a repeating cycle over the centuries. But change is in the air...

With the rise of information storage systems over hundreds of years, knowledge of all kinds has become much more accessible to millions of people around the world, including spiritual knowledge. What used to be transmitted orally from generation to generation became available in writings on stone and parchment. Then printed in books, which gave rise to an explosion of knowledge during the last millennium, and especially over the last few centuries. And now information is stored electronically on computers and beamed around the world instantly via the internet. The staying power of knowledge has greatly increased, and this is leading steadily to better application of all kinds of knowledge, including knowledge about how to maximize the inner capabilities of the human nervous system – opening our door to the infinite.

Yoga – Ancient and Ever-New

One of the oldest systems of knowledge designed for unfolding human spiritual potential is called *Yoga*, which means, "union" or "to join." That is union of the inner and outer qualities of life – opening the door of the human body and its inner circuitry, the nervous system, to its full latent potential. Yoga is not a religious system, though it can be and sometimes is combined with religion, mainly because people need a framework of belief to wrap around human spiritual experiences. The spiritual experiences cultivated by yoga practices are self-evident, with or without an attending belief system, in the same way spontaneous experiences of inner expansion are self-evident. The difference between spontaneous experiences and those cultivated by yoga is that the latter are systematic and lasting. This is what we would like, yes?

Everywhere around the world, yoga is thought to be primarily a system of physical postures and exercises for improving our health and well-being. That it is. Yet, yoga is much more than that. In fact, in the overall scheme of yoga, as described in the ancient *Yoga Sutras of Patanjali*, physical postures represent one of the eight limbs of yoga. Only one of eight. The other limbs are concerned with conduct, breathing practices, introversion of sensory perception, and powerful mental techniques that bring our divine inner qualities out into everyday living.

In this book we are covering the physical side of yoga in a way that can be linked up and integrated with the full capabilities of a broad-based system of yoga practices.

No one aspect of yoga stands alone, though there is a great temptation to believe that this is so. If we look around the world today, there are millions who are practicing yoga postures with great dedication. Likewise, there are those who are practicing breathing techniques with fervor, and others who are doing the same with meditation. In all cases, people are finding positive results that bring some peace and happiness into daily living. That is why people do the practices, sometimes going to great lengths to get the most out of a single aspect of practice.

But, in approaching it through a single class of practices, we are not likely to find the full unfoldment that yoga promises to deliver. That is because yoga is not a single-pronged strategy for opening the door of the human nervous system to the great potential we all have for peace, energy, creativity and divine unfoldment from within. Yoga is a multi-pronged system. For full success, all the aspects of yoga must be applied in a logical sequence, gradually built up and integrated over time.

Where does yoga come from in the first place? It comes from within us – from the underlying principles of spiritual transformation that are contained in each of us. So, yoga is not a system coming from outside us that we are reliant upon to open us to our greater possibilities. Yoga is a system that reflects our own inner capabilities – it is a mirror of who we are inside and how we naturally evolve to higher stages of functioning. This is the great difference between yoga and intermediary approaches to spiritual development. Yoga is a path that involves cultivating self-sufficiency on our spiritual path from the beginning, no matter which practices we happen to start with. Of course, there is a system of structured knowledge and logical orders of implementation according to particular teachings. Education is available to aid the journey. In that spirit, we will offer many suggestions here while delving into the physical practices of yoga.

Yoga is as relevant and new today as it was 5,000 years ago. Why? Because the human nervous system has not changed, and higher experience is as accessible now as it was then. Perhaps more so now, because knowledge of the methods for accelerating the process of human spiritual transformation has evolved steadily over the centuries, and in modern times has achieved a level of integration and efficiency that has not been seen before. What was complicated and difficult in the past has become straight forward and relatively easy. All it takes is a desire, consistent practice of tried and true methods, and the results will be readily apparent.

Asanas, Mudras & Bandhas to Join Body & Spirit

There are layers that constitute our physical and non-physical existence, and the methods of yoga are geared toward activating the principles of evolution operating at each layer – on each level of functioning within us. On the physical level, there is much we can do.

As implied by the title of this book, there is a logical division between physical practices:

Asanas – Postures, positions and seats we gently cultivate to improve the overall spiritual conductivity of our nervous system, especially the central spinal nerve.

<u>Mudras</u> – Physical, sometimes dynamic, positions focused on particular areas of the body that *seal* or channel the flow of neurobiological energies within us.

<u>Bandhas</u> – Physical, usually static, positions focused on particular areas of the body that *block* the flow of neurobiological energies within us, resulting in increased energy flow in the opposite direction.

Of these three, asanas are the best known by far. In fact, yoga postures have become an important part of the vast worldwide physical fitness industry. Yoga classes are available everywhere, and people are joining them in droves for the well-recognized relaxation and health benefits. The word "yoga" has become synonymous with physical postures in modern society, which is a narrow view, of course. Nevertheless, the popularity of yoga postures is a good thing. Once practitioners get a taste of the benefits that come from yoga postures, it is natural to look to the broader scope of yoga methods that are available, ultimately leading many to deep meditation, pranayama (breathing techniques), mudras, bandhas, and other practices comprising the multi-limbed tree of yoga. Ultimately, asanas are found to be an excellent limbering up that aids other yoga practices in taking the practitioner deep into the subtle strata of the nervous system, through the door to the infinite realm of pure bliss consciousness – our own eternal inner silence. This journey, taken each day, can produce profound effects in our daily living.

Mudras and bandhas, while classified as separate practices, have much similarity and overlap. These are physical maneuvers we can undertake, in conjunction with breathing practices and other methods, which influence the inner functioning of our nervous system. Mudras and bandhas are more inward in both performance and appearance, and tend to disappear entirely as visible practices in later stages of yoga where the natural manipulations of ecstatic energy in the nervous system become very subtle and automatic. In other words, mudras and bandhas are a gentle training of natural physical processes *within* the human body. Once these processes take over, the mudras and bandhas, while still performed in gross physical form in the practice routine, will also arise within the body with the advent of what we call *ecstatic conductivity*, or the awakening of *Kundalini*. In Christian terms it is the arrival of the *Holy Spirit*. However we may name the rise of spiritual ecstasy in the human body, and the vast creative power that comes with it, we will find the mudras and bandhas to be in the midst of it. Indeed, they are the natural outcome of an evolving nervous system, as are all the practices of yoga. We are only helping the process of evolution along by learning to encourage these inherent capabilities within us.

Just as there are overlaps between mudras and bandhas in both name and function, there are also overlaps between asanas, mudras and bandhas. This will become clear in the following chapters, where some of the overlaps will be pointed out. It is all one process of human spiritual transformation. The only reason it is divided up into categories of practice is so we can get our arms around it and engage in the practical application of effective techniques that will hasten our evolution. This is the genius of yoga.

Asanas, mudras and bandhas are primary means by which body and spirit are joined.

Going Beyond Relaxation

While most of us can use some relief from the stresses and strains of daily life, there is so much more we are capable of experiencing, if we choose to. The methods of yoga can bring some immediate relief for sure. It is one of the practical benefits of doing yoga practices. This sort of practicality can be taken much further. If we decide to travel the path of a broader application of practices, yoga can aid us in reaching far beyond what we might have imagined the quality of our life could be.

There is so much talk about *enlightenment* these days. Everyone wants to be enlightened. What on earth is it? There are so many definitions, both philosophical and experiential. We prefer the experiential. Why sit around talking about enlightenment when we can actually do something that will give an experience of it? And what is that?

To be happy. Not just happy for the moment, or for a while, but for all time – in sickness and in health until death do us part, as they say.

What do we mean by *happy*? Well, for starters, to be at peace with things as they are, no matter how they are. This does not mean passive or indifferent, like not sweeping the dirty sidewalk because we are happy with it just the way it is. We can be happy with the dirty sidewalk, we can be happy sweeping it, we can be happy with it when it is clean, and we can be happy with it when it is dirty again, and so on.

We can be active in the world, no longer traveling the cycle from misery to happiness and back to misery again, which has been the common experience of people for so many centuries. For certain, the ups and downs of life will always be there, but we will suffer much less as our inner functioning and perception evolve toward a more enlightened view.

We can be happy and act for the sake of acting, because the acting itself becomes a joy. But before we can do this, we must establish the connection with our inner nature, which is stillness and stirring ecstasy. It requires the application of a range of yoga techniques, some covered in this book, and others elsewhere in the AYP family of books. In pursuing the path of yoga, we will begin to witness the world like a movie, as separate from our sense of self. In that condition of *silent witness*, our awareness and desires will begin to inhabit the movie of the world in an increasing flow of love coming from inside, and in a flow of intentions and actions born from that divine quality being unleashed within us.

Yoga practices are for cultivating this condition in us – to open our inner door to the infinite that resides within. As the door is opened over time, we become imbued with unshakable inner silence, ecstatic bliss, and outpouring divine love. It is unending happiness, creativity, strength, and the ability to act harmoniously in every situation. This is not a guarantee of ultimate perfection, only a direction we can take that leads us toward more happiness in our daily living. If there is such a thing as enlightenment, then this is *It*.

Now let's take a look at the practical methods of asanas, mudras and bandhas in relation to an overall routine of yoga practices, and see how these can help us move along our path toward more happiness in daily living.

Chapter 2 – Asanas

There is something of a paradox here. The teaching and practice of asanas (yoga postures) is a huge worldwide phenomenon. It has moved over into the mainstream of the physical fitness industry, with numerous kinds of aerobic and extreme yoga regimens now available. This is big business!

Yet, in the overall scheme of traditional yoga, asanas are only one limb out of eight, with meditation, pranayama and the other limbs having equal or greater weight. Not to mention the important tri-limbed practice of samyama, which expands the influence of inner silence in all aspects of life.

Why the difference between the basic truths of full scope yoga practice and what we see going on in the world? Some say it is "market driven." We are a culture that craves physical health above all things. It is understandable. We all want our health and well-being, the more the better.

But learning to systematically do less can be much more, you know. That is the secret of yoga. In the AYP approach to yoga practices we use asanas primarily as a limbering, a stretching of the nervous system to warm up for spinal breathing pranayama, deep meditation and other *sitting practices*.

Postures - An Important Limb of Yoga

Asanas, or physical postures, are important in any approach to yoga, no matter where we have started – with pranayama, with meditation, with devotional activity, or even with studies of the philosophical side of yoga. Of course, these days, many people start with asanas, so it is very often not a case of adding asana practice, but adding the rest of yoga! Either way, we will be wise to consider the full range of practices available from the ancient wisdom of yoga in order to achieve the best results. This does not mean adding more and more yoga postures and time duration until the time we are doing postures each day runs into hours, squeezing everything else out. It is a much more refined, balanced and efficient process of yoga we are seeking.

What we will find is that if we develop a range of both postures and sitting practices step-by-step in a well-integrated way, then each part can be kept to a reasonable time with *increased effectiveness* of the overall routine. With that, we can accomplish more with less, and still have plenty of time to go out into our daily activities and enjoy the benefits. That is the payoff for any kind of yoga practice, yes? Enhancement in the quality of our life, as we choose to live it.

The approach suggested in this book is two short sets of asanas each day, morning and evening, followed by our sitting practices, which include spinal breathing pranayama, deep meditation, samyama, mudras and bandhas (covered in the next chapter), and other techniques.

The fact that yoga postures have caught on with the public cannot be denied. Much good comes from it. It doesn't matter which limb of yoga caught on first. All the limbs of yoga are connected. If we do asanas, we will be drawn to pranayama and meditation eventually. If we do meditation, we will be drawn to asanas eventually. That is how it goes. Our nervous system knows a good thing when it sees it. Wake up the nervous system a little and it wants more. All of the limbs of yoga are expressions of the natural ways that our nervous system opens to divine experience.

Our nervous system determines the practices, not the other way around. Practices come to us when we need them. It is amazing how this happens. It is the power of our desire for evolution that brings knowledge to us. When this desire is sustained, it is called *bhakti*. In time, all of the practices come together automatically. We just have to give a nudge here and there. That is the power of bhakti.

We live in a world where human experience is based mainly on physicality. Our senses are yet to be drawn inward to the point where inner experiences will become as real (or more real) than experiences in the external world. So we are always looking for a physical solution. Yoga asanas begin to take us from physicality to more subtle experiences of divine energy in the nervous system. This is why asanas are so relaxing. It is their main draw. People do asanas for relaxation, for some inner peace. Yoga asanas are very good for that. They are also very good for preparing the body and mind for pranayama and meditation. This is the way we will look at asanas here – as a preparation in our daily routine for pranayama and meditation.

There are exceptions to the "relaxing" mode of asanas. Nowadays, you can go take a class in power yoga, aerobic yoga, and get a good workout. That is okay. It is not suggested for right before pranayama and meditation though. We are going the other way when we go into sitting practices, to less activity in the nervous system, not more. So we do our aerobic activities after our yoga routine, not right before it.

The physical conditioning aspect of life is not ignored here – it is very important, especially for those whose ecstatic energies have been awakened. For a yoga-friendly routine of muscle toning calisthenics and aerobic (cardiovascular) development, see the appendix at the end of the book.

Asanas in the traditional sense are for quieting the nervous system. But more than that. They are designed to facilitate the flow of *prana* (life force) in the body, particularly in the *sushumna*, which is the central spinal nerve. So you can see that asanas are a natural preparation for pranayama, particularly spinal breathing pranayama.

Asanas are part of a broader system of primarily physical yoga called *hatha yoga*. In hatha yoga, there are also the mudras and bandhas, which are targeted approaches to moving prana in the body. There is an Indian scripture called the *Hatha Yoga Pradipika* that covers both asanas and mudras and bandhas. Many of the physical yoga practices in use today can be found in this ancient book. The practices can be found in other systems as well, such as in *kundalini yoga* and in *tantra yoga*. Many systems of yoga utilize asanas, mudras and bandhas. There is a lot of overlap. Everyone wants to lay claim to a good thing.

It all comes down to what works, and each system of yoga is seeking to achieve best results in its own way. That is the mission of AYP also, except it is open to the general public, rather than reserved for a few selected practitioners.

Hatha yoga means "joining of the sun and the moon" – joining the masculine and feminine energies within us. We run into this theme in every tradition, because it is an essential characteristic of an evolving human nervous system. In India it is also known as the joining of the metaphorical Kundalini-Shakti and Shiva within us. Kundalini-Shakti is the ecstatic aspect of our inner functioning, awakened by asanas, mudras, bandhas and pranayama, while Shiva represents the emergence of blissful inner silence within us, awakened in deep meditation and samyama. The Taoists represent this duality with Yin and Yang. The Christians call them the Holy Spirit and God the Father. And so on…

No matter what tradition we find ourselves in, the operation of the nervous system will be the same as it evolves to higher stages of functioning. Only the names may be different.

As they say, "A rose is still a rose by any other name."

There is some overlap between asanas and the mudras and bandhas. Some yoga practices keep the name *asana;* others might carry the name *mudra* or *bandha.* Whatever we call them, they are physical practices facilitating the movement of prana and blissful inner silence within us. So, when you see *yoga mudra* and *maha mudra* in the asana list, and *siddhasana* in the mudra and bandha list, do not be surprised. Such overlaps are not uncommon. The most important thing is that we are applying these methods in the most effective manner in relation to the sequence and duration of our practices.

Asana Starter Kit

There are many ways to learn how to do asanas (classes, videos, books), and many styles out there to choose from. Here in this book, we will make it very easy. We are going to introduce fourteen simple postures to do before our sitting practices. *Simple* is a good place to start, yes? We will call it our *Asana Starter Kit.*

No doubt there will be some who want more.

Plenty more is available. With thousands of yoga teachers around the world, and dozens of systems of practice, the possibilities for yoga posture training are practically endless.

Our goal here is to establish a phase-in for our sitting practices of spinal breathing pranayama, meditation, and so on. For those who are looking for a place to start with asanas, this book can suffice. It will be very simple.

Surely many reading here will already have a class in yoga asanas under their belt – maybe a lot of classes. That is good. Taking a yoga class is highly recommended, as long as it is the slow and easy variety of asanas that are conducive for pranayama and meditation right afterward. See the appendix for a discussion of aerobic exercise.

For those who are into yoga postures already, this will be a review, and perhaps even a *toning down* from an expanding routine of postures that may take an increasingly large chunk of time out of the day. It has been found to be much more effective to add sitting practices at the end of a modest asana routine than to keep increasing the asana routine without the addition of sitting practices. In fact, the asana routine can be shortened, while increasing the overall effect with a combined routine involving sitting practices.

There are many ways to approach it, depending on one's background, training and inclination. But one thing is for sure. Asanas, pranayama and meditation, in balanced proportion time-wise, make a far more effective routine of practice than asanas alone. So that is the angle we are coming from here.

With that, let's take a look at the basic asana routine. The routine can be done in about ten minutes right before pranayama and meditation. Illustrations for the postures are included. We will also provide an abbreviated routine of just a few minutes for those who are on the go, the rationale being that, when there is a schedule pinch, it is preferable to spend most of our limited practice time doing meditation and pranayama.

We will look at fourteen basic postures here, which are done on the floor. If you have a mat, great, but there's no need to run out and buy one. A soft carpet with a large towel or blanket laid out will do just fine for this routine. Make sure you have your comfortable meditation clothing on before you start.

It is important that you not force any of these postures. If the posture calls for a toe touch and you can only reach your shin comfortably, stop there. That is the perfect posture for you. Never strain in a posture. In fact, that is the rule for all yoga practices. It is the essence of personal *self-pacing* in practices, which is at the heart of all progress in yoga. Here is the routine:

1. **Heart Centering Warm-up** – Sit on the floor cross-legged. Gently massage your head with both hands as you move your hands down toward your heart – first down the front of your face and neck to your heart, and then down the back of your head and around your neck and down the front to your heart. Those two movements can be done in 15 seconds or so. Not too fast and not too slow. Now do the same thing with the left arm, starting with the left hand, using the right hand to gently massage all the way back to the heart – first along the top of the arm, over the shoulder and down the chest to the heart, and then along

the bottom side of the arm, through the arm pit
and to the heart. The left arm is done with the
right hand like that. Now switch to the right arm
and do it with the left hand the same way. Now do
both legs from the toes all the way up to the heart
– just a gentle moving two-handed massage on
each leg. As you come up from each leg press in
gently on your belly and solar plexus region with
both hands on the way up to the heart. Finally,
reach in back with both hands and do one moving
massage from the buttocks, up your back and
around to your chest and heart. All of these heart
centering warm-up movements can be done in a
minute or so. If you are wondering what to do
with your attention during this heart centering,
just let it be easy, going with your hands as they
gently massage your energy toward your heart.
Let your breathing be easy also. This is how we
handle attention and breathing in all these basic
postures, easy and relaxed with whatever we are
doing physically, unless instructed otherwise.

2. **Knees to Chest Roll** – Lie on your back and
bring your knees up far enough so you can grasp
each upper shin with each hand. Or, if you can
reach, clasp you fingers together around your
upper shins, near the knees. Let your knees come
toward your chest. Now roll from side to side,
about five times each way, right to left, letting
your head roll from side to side on the floor along
with your torso. Roll as far to each side as is
comfortable.

3. **Kneeling Seat** (Vajrasana) – Get up straight on
your knees with legs nearly together. Put one big

toe over the other behind you, and then sit down on your heels, keeping your torso up straight. Let your hands rest on your thighs or in your lap. Sit like this for about 10 seconds. (Use a mental count until you get a good feel for the 10-second hold on all of these postures.) Then go up straight on your knees again for a few seconds and back down into the seat for another 10 seconds. Go up again, and then relax. Sit on the floor with your feet in front of you.

4. **Sitting Head to Knee** (Janushirshasana and Paschimottanasana) – While sitting, put your left leg out straight and bring your right foot in toward your crotch. If it will go comfortably all the way, then let your right heel rest against your perineum. If the right foot won't go all the way in to the crotch, then just let it rest however far inward it will go with comfort. Now lean forward while extending your hands toward your left foot. If you can reach, then grab your left big toe with both hands. If you can't reach your toe, then just let your hands rest on your left shin however far you can comfortably go. Let your torso and head come down as far as comfortable. If you are very limber, your head may end up resting on your left knee. If it won't go that far, then just stop at your comfortable limit as you lean forward. Hold that position for about 10 seconds. Now reverse the whole thing and do it with your right leg extended and your left leg in toward your crotch. Hold it again for 10 seconds. Finally, do it with both legs out straight. This time, grab your left and right toes with your left and right hands, respectively. Or, if you can't reach, just let each hand rest on

its corresponding shin at your comfortable limit of stretch. As with the other head to knee positions, let your torso and head come down toward your knees to a comfortable limit, and hold for about 10 seconds. Then relax. A more advanced version of the left and right head to knee posture involves sitting up on the heel, putting more pressure on the perineum, and holding a full breath inside while doing the posture. This advanced version of head to knee is called *Maha Mudra*, and it is described in more detail in the next chapter.

5. **Shoulder Stand** (Viparitakarani or Sarvangasana) – Lie on your back with your hands at your sides. Bring your knees up and roll your buttocks up in the air, while bringing your hands under your upward curling back. Keep going up and straighten your legs and back out above you. Use your hands to support your back by propping them up with your elbows on the floor. Find a comfortable balance in this posture, and hold for about 10 seconds. It doesn't have to be straight up. The idea is to achieve inversion of your body. That is the main purpose of the shoulder stand. Before you come back down, go to the next posture.

6. **Plow** (Halasana) – While in the shoulder stand, let your legs and torso come down over your head, going toward the floor. Continue to support your back with your hands with elbows on the floor, as necessary. If you can, let your feet come all the way down to the floor with your legs straight, and let your arms down to lie flat on the floor behind you. Hold this posture for about 10

seconds. If the legs and back will not come far enough to let your feet touch the floor, then stop at your comfortable limit. In that case you can let your knees bend toward your shoulders for comfort, as if you are curling into a ball while propped up on your shoulder blades with your arms supporting your back as in the shoulder stand. If you end up in that curled up position, hold it for about 10 seconds. Whichever degree of the plow you come to, after the 10 second hold, uncurl yourself gently back down to lying flat on your back with your hands at your sides.

7. **Seal of Yoga** (Yoga Mudra) – Sit on the floor cross-legged. Clasp your hands comfortably behind your back with arms hanging loose. Lean forward with your head and torso to your comfortable limit. If you are limber, your head may touch the floor. Hold this posture at your comfortable limit for about 10 seconds, and then sit back up.

8. **Cobra** (Bhujangasana) – Roll over onto your stomach, lying flat on the floor. Put your hands under your shoulders as if you are going to do a push-up. Lift your head and shoulders up using your upper back, with a little help from your arms. Your belly should not leave the floor. You will have a good arch in your back. Hold this posture for about 10 seconds, and come back down gently.

9. **Locust** (Shalabhasana) – Still on your stomach, lying flat on the floor, extend your arms with both hands, palms up, under both sides of your pelvis.

Keeping your legs straight, lift your knees up using your lower back. Hold this posture for about 10 seconds, and come back down gently.

10. **Spinal Twist** (Ardha Matsyendrasana) – Sit on the floor with your right leg out straight. Place your left foot on the floor just outside your right knee. Your left knee will be sticking up in front of you. Reach with your right arm past the left side of your left knee and use your elbow against the knee to twist your torso to the left. With your left arm, reach around behind you, further twisting your torso to the left, and touch the floor behind you with your left hand. Turn your head to the left also, looking as far around to the left as you can. Hold this twist for about 10 seconds. Don't strain in the twist. Only twist as far around as is comfortable. Now, switch legs and do the same posture the other way, twisting to the right, again holding for about 10 seconds. Then relax.

11. **Abdominal Lift** (Uddiyana Bandha) – Stand up, with feet shoulder-width apart, leaning with your hands on your knees. Take a deep breath and expel as much air from your lungs as you can. With air expelled, suck your belly in and up using your diaphragm. Hold your belly in and up like that for about five seconds, and then release your belly, but do not breathe in yet. Pull the belly in and up again for five seconds. And again for five seconds more. Now relax and take a deep breath. This posture is called uddiyana bandha. It can also be practiced in an advanced variation called *Nauli*. This is covered in the uddiyana bandha discussion in the next chapter.

12. **Standing Back Stretch** (Urdhvasana) – Standing with feet a little apart, reach with your straightened arms over your head and back as far as you comfortably can. Bend back with your spine as you do this, being careful not to fall over backwards. Hold this posture for about 10 seconds. Then stand up straight again and relax.

13. **Standing Toe Touch** (Padahastasana)– Standing with feet a little apart, reach down toward the floor with your hands while keeping your knees straight. Touch or grab your toes if you can without discomfort. If you are limber, you can let your palms rest flat on the floor. In doing this posture, your head may come close to your knees, or even touch them. If you can't reach, that is okay. Let your hands and head come down to whatever your comfortable limit is. Hold this posture for about 10 seconds.

14. **Corpse Pose** (Shavasana) – Lie down on your back with arms and legs spread a little, and relax. Let your mind relax completely. Remain in this posture for about one minute. Longer if you like. Now you are ready to take your seat for pranayama and meditation.

All of these postures can be done in about 10 minutes. If you are in a hurry, you can do them in less time, but that is not recommended.

These are basic asanas, and most of them can be performed in more advanced versions. Nauli, an advanced version of uddiyana is covered in the next chapter on mudras and bandhas. It is very good for stimulating a higher form of digestion. Maha mudra, also covered in the next chapter, is an advanced version of the head to knee posture for those who are ready to incorporate breath retention and several mudras and bandhas into a single posture. Maha mudra is an excellent way to loosen up the sushumna before pranayama and meditation, and to aid in awakening the inner ecstatic energies.

There are additional enhancements that can be worked into the asana routine over time, according to personal preference. This is a basic routine – a starter kit. It is suitable to prepare the nervous system for sitting practices.

Abbreviated Asana Starter Kit

For those who are short on time, there is still the opportunity to do some limbering up before sitting practices. The trick is to do some twisting, abdominal lift, backward bending, forward bending and inversion. These are the essential elements that lie at the core of most asanas. Together, they flex and manipulate the spinal nerve, preparing it for spinal breathing and deep meditation. For that purpose, the following abbreviated all-standing routine is offered that can be done in a couple of minutes.

1. **Standing Spinal Twist** – Stand with feet shoulder-width apart and reach around behind you to the left as far as you can with both arms wrapping around your torso in that direction. Let your torso and head twist in that direction as far as comfortable. Hold this posture for about 10 seconds. Relax, and then do it in the other direction.

2. **Abdominal Lift** – Stand with feet apart and do

this the same as described in #11 above.

3. **Standing Back Stretch** – Stand with feet a little apart, and do this posture the same as described in #12 above.

4. **Standing Toe Touch** – Stand with feet a little apart, and do this posture the same as described in #13 above. Besides flexing the spinal nerve forward, this posture also provides inversion, though not to the same degree as a shoulder stand.

From here you can go straight into your sitting practices. If you have the time and space to lie down for a minute (corpse pose) before beginning pranayama, that is good too. These four postures can be compressed down into a minute or so if time is very short, or stretched out to several minutes. If there is not enough time for a full set of asanas, this abbreviated session will be much better than no asanas. It does not require getting down on the floor, and can be done in street clothes just about anywhere.

Illustrations for the Asana Starter Kit are provided on the following pages. In time, you may tend toward more advanced versions of these, and add more postures into the mix. Or you may stick with this routine. Either way, you have this starter routine and can do some good bending and stretching that will aid you in settling into your sitting practices.

1a. Warm-up, head to heart   1b. Warm-up, arms to heart   1c. Warm-up, legs to heart

 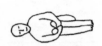

2a. Knees to chest   2b. Roll, right then left   3. Kneeling seat

 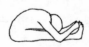 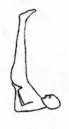

4a. Sitting, head to one knee   4b. Sitting, head to both knees   5. Shoulder stand

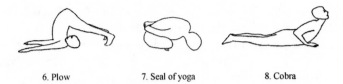

6. Plow   7. Seal of yoga   8. Cobra

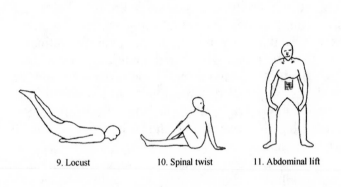

9. Locust   10. Spinal twist   11. Abdominal lift

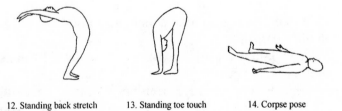

12. Standing back stretch   13. Standing toe touch   14. Corpse pose

Practice Routines and Self-Pacing

Now that we have looked at a basic routine of asanas, let's look closer at its implementation in relation to our overall practice routine.

"But asanas *are* my overall practice routine!" you say.

Well, that has been fine until now, but do you really want to continue driving around in a car with only one wheel? No matter how big that wheel is, it will still be only one wheel. With that being the situation, the most important thing we can say about asanas is that they belong in an overall routine of practices that includes spinal breathing pranayama, deep meditation, mudras and bandhas, and even more methods of practice. Unfortunately, space does not permit full coverage of all these techniques here. But everything is covered in the full range of AYP writings that are available.

For now, we will focus on asanas (plus mudras and bandhas in the next chapter), and how these fit into an overall practice routine. The resulting effects will be reviewed and self-pacing for progress and safety will be discussed.

The Ideal Practice Routine

What is the ideal practice routine? Interestingly, what may be ideal for one person may not be ideal for another person.

You know the old saying, "One man's meat is another man's poison."

That is why we say, "routines." Plural. To each, his or her own. But there is a basic structure, you know. It is not just, *anything goes*. What we seek in our routine is a balance that is not over-weighted or under-weighted in any particular practice, or class of practices, such as asanas.

Now maybe some who are reading this are doing an hour or more of asanas every day – maybe for years. That is fine. But by the time we add deep meditation, spinal breathing pranayama and a few other things, that one hour of asanas may begin to feel pretty top-heavy. Maybe it is top-heavy already, and that is why a broader, more streamlined, approach to yoga practices is being suggested. Either way, there are practical realities to deal with in building a solid practice routine. In doing so, an excess in any particular area of practice will likely be trimmed, by necessity, because to not do so will likely lead to ongoing discomfort. Who wants that?

Obviously, we are talking about much more than *relaxation* here. We are talking about cultivating a permanent change in the inner functioning of our neurobiology that will bring us steadily into an experience of life that transcends what we have known so far – abiding inner silence, ecstatic bliss and outpouring divine love! To move beyond relaxation to enlightenment, a more sophisticated approach than one method (or one limb of yoga) will be necessary. It takes an integration of effective practices to get the job done. This is the key to success in yoga. Not necessarily more and more asanas, more and more meditation, or more and more pranayama. But, instead, more and more integration of methods across the limbs of yoga.

So, what is the ideal practice routine?

It is the balancing of whatever practices we are doing. If we are coming in with an hour of asanas, we might consider dropping back to a half hour of asanas and adding twenty minutes of deep meditation, with five or ten minutes of rest at the end. This simple modification will likely be far more powerful than the original hour of asanas was. It may be too powerful. So then we can back off the asanas some more. Or maybe we will decide to back off on meditation a bit to fifteen minutes, and see how that is. By trial and error, we can find our ideal routine.

Then, in a few weeks or months, we may be getting inspired and want to add another practice – spinal breathing pranayama is next on the list. So we do that, starting with five minutes, and the balancing act begins all over again. And so on we go in building our integrated practice routine.

It should be added that we are talking about a twice-daily routine here – once before breakfast, and again before the evening meal. This is particularly important for deep meditation and spinal breathing pranayama, in order to maintain the inner momentum of purification and opening around the clock. It is a cycle of going inward during sitting practices, followed by activity, twice each day. This is optimal for stabilizing the benefits of yoga practice.

If we are coming to all of this for the first time, it is a good. We will have few preconceived notions. Then we can take on practices in an order that will bring the most results the soonest, with emphasis on comfort and safety. In that case, we can pick up deep meditation first, then spinal breathing pranayama, then asanas, then mudras and bandhas after that, and so on. It can take years to build it up. Or we may only go as far as deep meditation, some light spinal breathing and asanas. These three make an excellent integrated routine.

What is the order and time of these practices?

It is just as we have mentioned before – asanas first (5-15 minutes), spinal breathing pranayama second (5-10 minutes), deep meditation third (15-20 minutes), and a period of rest at the end (5-10 minutes, lying down in corpse pose, if desired). That is an excellent routine that can be done before the morning and evening meal, taking from 30 minutes to an hour for each session, according to how long we are doing each practice. This is a routine that can make a huge difference in our everyday activities in the world, as we see ourselves moving steadily beyond relaxation to something much more – the steady rise of inner silence, peace, creativity and joy in all that we do.

As we will see later on, mudras and bandhas add little to our time of practice, while adding a lot in results. They are largely overlapped in time with the practices already mentioned. So, time-wise, mudras and bandhas are a bonus. A big bonus, considering the extent to which they can enhance the effects of all of our practices and put us on the road to the safe awakening of our ecstatic inner nature, also called *kundalini*.

Purification of the Neurobiology

We have mentioned the importance of not straining, and self-pacing of our practices to sustain good progress in yoga with safety. What is it that we mean by all this? If we are doing some bending and stretching, some breathing exercises, and some meditation, how could any of these be hazardous? Sure, we can see that over-reaching in a posture could strain a muscle or tendon, but what do we mean by changing the inner functioning of our neurobiology?

This highlights a fundamental principle in yoga – the *gradual cultivation* of higher functioning. Nothing in yoga is a sprint. It is a marathon from beginning to end. Whenever we try and go fast and hard in yoga, we will be risking excessive purification, injury, and delays. This applies not only to the obvious physical aspects we find in asanas, but also to the inner aspects that are influenced by mudras, bandhas, spinal breathing pranayama, and deep meditation.

Asanas provide a good example of what is involved. The degree of comfortable stretch we can do in a posture right now is the ideal posture for us today. If we are leaning over to touch our toes and can only reach comfortably to our shins, then that is the perfect execution of that posture. If we are doing our asana routine twice daily, in a few weeks or months, we may find that our comfortable reach has gone down the shin, maybe even to the ankles. In six months or a year, maybe to our feet. It all depends on the change going on in the muscles, tendons and nerves. All three are involved in yoga postures. It is a gradual cultivation that brings us slowly but steadily toward greater flexibility, relaxation and inner opening. Of course, we may be doing other yoga practices as well, and perhaps moving toward a purer lifestyle that will add to our physical flexibility and inner purification. All of these things work together. Remember, success in yoga comes from an integration of methods.

When it comes to the nervous system, things get much more subtle. Asanas help our nerves to become more flexible and less stressed. Spinal breathing pranayama acts directly on the nervous system, and so does deep meditation at the most subtle level within us. With pranayama and meditation we are working on levels of the nervous system that are less physical, taking us steadily beyond the obvious relaxation that postures bring. With asanas, we begin the relaxation process. With spinal breathing and deep meditation, we take it much deeper. This leads to purification of the nervous system in ways that enhance the flow of the life force within us – or *prana*. The purer the nervous system, the better the flow of life force within us. And, hence, more inner silence, more peace, more creativity, more joy and so on. It is purification of the neurobiology that brings about all these positive changes. So, first and foremost, yoga and all of its methods constitute a process of purification in our nervous system. It is by this that all the good results of yoga are experienced, from basic relaxation, onward to full-blown enlightenment for the person who travels the path with persistence and good pacing of practices.

The purification of the neurobiology is a long term, delicate process. The analogy of flushing out dirty pipes has been used, and this is one way to look at it. However, there is a widely held misconception that this can be done very quickly – blasting away the obstructions in the nervous system virtually overnight. It would be nice, but that is not the reality experienced by many serious practitioners of yoga. Whether one is practicing a few months or a few decades, the process is ongoing – a long journey of purification and opening within, with steady progress month after month, and year after year. On it goes.

The very best systems of yoga are those that promote this process on the edge of too much purification, allowing the practitioner to press onward without pressing beyond their limits. There are many tell-tale experiences along the way, which indicate the process of purification and opening is occurring. A seasoned practitioner knows that each new experience is but a signpost along the highway leading toward enlightenment. And so they go on, never proclaiming arrival until, finally, there is no need to.

Enlightenment is not an arrival after all, but a natural and complete letting go of that which has been sought. It is not a decision or a revelation, but a state of being that gradually emerges in the yoga practitioner, bit by bit, as the neurobiology is purified. In the end, there is nothing but peace, joy, and serving for the benefit of others. It is our birthright.

How to Avoid Excess and Strain

The first rule in all yoga practices is to never force, and always use gentle persuasion. In the case of postures, if there is some stiffness, injury, or discomfort, then we just go to our natural limit and test it a little. Never to the point of pain or strain. Just to the point of the limit of movement, and then be there for the time of our posture. This may be nowhere near the full expression of the posture, which is perfectly fine. We do what we can comfortably in the direction of the posture without strain, knowing we will be doing gradually more in subsequent sessions. If any degree of stretch becomes uncomfortable, we back off to a comfortable level. Or, if it can go a little further without strain, then we let it. It is the principle of *self-pacing* applied in postures. This is the fine art of progressing in yoga – never forcing, always using gentle persuasion, and always backing off when it is too much. With this approach, the body and nervous system slowly but surely move to more flexibility, purification and greater experiences of inner peace and bliss.

There is an old saying, "By the yard, life is hard. By the inch, it's a cinch." It is easy to become advanced in any aspect of yoga practice if we know how to handle self-pacing.

Overdoing in Asanas

If we have been inclined to be doing long routines of postures, like an hour or more, and we have come to that level quickly without a gradual buildup over weeks and months, then there is the risk of overdoing and having discomfort after our practice. Why? Because asanas will loosen obstructions in our nervous system just as most yoga practices will. If this is done to excess at a given point in time, there will be some "grinding of the gears" in the nervous system, which can be experienced as physical or emotional discomfort. Then we will be faced with the task of bringing the purification going on within us back into balance, which can take some time. So the best thing is to not overdo in the first place.

If such symptoms occur after our asana routine, and it is not from overdoing, then maybe we did not rest long enough (in corpse pose) at the end of our routine and something went out of balance from getting up too soon instead of being released during practice and rest. This is assuming an asana routine that is not followed by spinal breathing pranayama and deep meditation.

Physical postures, when taken alone and to excess, are more likely to cause discomfort (especially emotional) than postures followed by spinal breathing pranayama and deep meditation. It is much better to do all of these three practices in sequence, and in moderation, with balanced purification occurring within. That is the approach we use here. A flexible guideline is 10 minutes asanas, 5 minutes pranayama, 20 minutes meditation, and 5-10 minutes rest twice each day. The times can be adjusted up or down to fit the individual via self-pacing.

Of course, prevention will not help us much once we have overdone it with asanas. As they say, "An ounce of prevention is worth a pound of cure."

If we have overdone, we just have to take some time to heal. And we will heal. First, we should be kind to ourselves, knowing that things will be all right again soon. We should back off practices, as necessary, until we feel stability of energy and emotions returning again. Some light spinal breathing and deep meditation can help. Taking long walks is an excellent way to balance the inner energies that have been thrown off temporarily. We will heal, and in the future will provide for moderation and balance our routine. Yoga is powerful stuff, and works well when done in correct proportions. Too much in the wrong combination can lead to trouble – too much purification too fast. It is just a matter of education, and prudent self-pacing according to experiences.

The reason we do yoga is because something in us wants to grow. We have a desire to engage in practices. Our ongoing desire for inner growth (bhakti) is good. It fuels practice. Of course, the tendency to overdo is the caution. There are many ways to overdo in yoga practices – as many ways as there are practices. Self-pacing has a lot of nuances to it. As we gain experience, we gradually become familiar with the terrain of our inner purification, and act according to the signals perceived along the way. We learn to trim practices temporarily at the first sign of excess purification. And in doing so, we are able to pick up again and move forward quickly, instead of spending days or weeks recovering from an overdose of inner energy flows.

With our ongoing desire to travel the path of purification and opening, and with wise self-pacing, we will be able to maximize our progress while maintaining good comfort and safety. There are many joys we will experience along the way.

Physical Exercise Before and After Yoga Practices

As discussed earlier, traditional yoga postures are for relaxing the nervous system in preparation for spinal breathing pranayama and deep meditation, which take us to progressively deeper levels of inner stillness. This stillness is the primary source of all spiritual progress. Asanas are part of this process of going to stillness. With easy bending and stretching we begin to loosen and quiet the nerves, and prepare the spinal nerve for pranayama. With pranayama, we further quiet our entire nervous system and cultivate it in a way that prepares it for deep meditation. That is the traditional sequence for best results in a routine of practices – asanas, pranayama and meditation. And it really does work.

In modern times, the application of yoga postures has been expanded to include physical fitness, including strenuous exercise designed to elevate the breathing, heart rate and cardiovascular activity. In other words, exercise. Like any other kind of vigorous exercise, yoga postures done in this way have value for our physical conditioning. However, this is not the style of yoga asana routine we should be doing right before we are going to sit to meditate. It is obviously going in the opposite direction – to more activity in the body, not less. If we wish to exercise, it will be wise to do it *after* our yoga practices which are for bringing us to inner stillness, or at least thirty minutes before them.

It is suggested to do the easy bending and stretching portion of asanas at the beginning, right before pranayama and meditation, so we can get the full benefit of the sequence. After meditation and adequate rest coming out, then it is a good time to do more vigorous physical exercise. See the appendix for more on an exercise program that is compatible with yoga.

So, first we do those things in the best order to take us in to pure bliss consciousness (our inner silence), and then we come out refreshed and ready to be active in the world. Vigorous activity after meditation is not a problem once we have taken time to come completely out. Activity helps stabilize the silent bliss and ecstasy in our nervous system. That is how we transform to become the walking enlightened, instead of the walking whatever we were before.

Movements and Automatic Yoga

Sometimes when we are meditating, there can be involuntary physical movements. They can come in the form of small jerks or even large movements, without our thinking about it. Such movements occurring now and then during practices are normal. It is energy opening inner neurobiological pathways. The movements will reduce as the inner pathways open and offer less resistance.

Sometimes movements point to *automatic yoga* positions. For example, if we feel compelled to go down to the mat with our head and torso while sitting in pranayama or meditation, this is the sushumna (spinal nerve) wanting to stretch itself for more purification (*yoga mudra*). If we happen to do some *maha mudra* and *yoga mudra* as part of our asanas before pranayama and meditation it can help pre-empt the tendency during sitting practices. If our head and torso irresistibly want to go down during sitting practices, then we let them for a few minutes, or we can let ourselves go into it for as long as necessary at the end of our sitting practices. It is a natural expression of the connectedness of yoga through our nervous system that is occurring.

Obviously, we don't want to interrupt our sitting practices too much with spontaneous yoga positions, but sometimes these things happen, so we let them if the urge becomes strong enough. One of the best ways to minimize movements in pranayama and meditation is with a good set of asanas before we start. Then the stretching has been initiated already and the body will be happy to go deep in pranayama and meditation.

If the movements become too much, we do as we always do when symptoms of purification become excessive. We use self-pacing in our practices and back off for a while until we find stability in our routine, and continue from there. When we hit a few potholes in the road, we slow down until the road smoothes out again.

The occasional jerks are common at certain stages of development, and a sign of purification going on – milestones on the road to enlightenment and more happiness in life.

Electric Jolts – What are They?

Another form of inner purification that can come during or after our asanas is an electric-like jolt surging suddenly through the body. It can be accompanied by strong euphoric emotions – a giddiness that lasts for several minutes or hours, which can be followed later on by sagging emotions in the aftermath of the experience.

The feeling of electricity is energy creating friction in our not yet fully purified nerves. The giddiness is from this also, as is the emotional let down that can come later on. Such surges are not common, but do happen – it is a classic kundalini surge.

Electric jolts are surely not an experience we want to have happening on an ongoing basis, even though it can have euphoric short-term effects. What we want is smooth and pleasant long term progress, always.

Chances are we have been pushing it with our practices for a few days or weeks before such experiences occur. The experience is a signal to lighten up a bit on practices until things smooth out. Then we can resume our normal yoga routine again.

We should always make sure to take plenty of rest coming out of our practices, and have good activity during the day and evening after practices – mental, physical, social, a good blend of these over the weeks and months. If we don't stabilize what we gain in practices with activity in the world, the stimulated inner energy can sometimes lurch through like that. Activity is an important part of the process of purification and the stabilization of inner silence and ecstatic energies we gain in practices.

A light to moderate set of asanas before sitting practices can help with stabilization, as can a diet that is neither too light nor too heavy. Moderation is valuable in all aspects of life, including yoga. With a little trial and error we will get the feel for our own process of unfoldment. Once we achieve self-sufficiency in regulating our practices in accordance with our experiences, then nothing can stop us from forging ahead safely and surely toward our goal.

Asanas in Relation to the Overall Yoga Program

One of the primary purposes of this book is to suggest balance between the various aspects of yoga in relation to asanas. If no asanas are being done in a daily routine of pranayama and meditation, then here can be a start for those who would like to move to a well-rounded program of practices. For those who are heavy into asanas, and little else on the tree of yoga, then the suggestion is to find balance by adding pranayama and meditation, while perhaps paring back on yoga postures if the routine has been excessive.

We have attempted to put asanas into perspective in relation to a full range of yoga practices as summarized in the *Yoga Sutras of Patanjali*. What we are seeking is a balance of all the best methods to achieve maximum progress.

There are thousands of skilled instructors teaching asanas around the world these days, and hundreds of excellent books and tapes on the subject. Yoga postures are well-covered. That is why we have not gone deeper here. However, the integration of postures into a thorough and well-balanced routine of yoga practices has been barely covered at all. Hence, this book.

How asanas fit into an overall system of yoga practices is a question that asana practitioners are asking these days. It is a good thing. Many who have gone heavily for yoga asanas often end up feeling that something is missing. As mentioned, in the AYP approach to yoga, asanas are a warm up for sitting practices. In other systems of practice, asanas may be an end in themselves, even though they represent only one-eighth of the traditional eight limbs of yoga. It is our culture, you know. It is changing, going more and more toward our inner divinity, and bringing *That* back out into the world through our daily activities becoming increasingly illuminated from within.

Activity in the physical world is essential for yoga to fulfill its destiny. Asanas help us on the way in, before we do our pranayama and deep meditation. When we are back out in the world, a healthy amount of physical activity and useful endeavors in our daily life are important. Both our sitting practices and daily activities in the world are what cultivate the steady-state condition of ecstatic bliss and divine love. Asanas have a special role to play in this – aiding the nervous system in its daily journey from outer activity inward to inner silence and ecstasy. In time, all of life becomes permeated with these inner divine qualities we are cultivating in our yoga practices.

Chapter 3 – Mudras and Bandhas

While asanas are well known, at least for their physical characteristics and general benefits to the public, mudras and bandhas are still most likely to be labeled *esoteric*, if they are recognized at all. By mudras and bandhas we mean the inner physical maneuvers we can systematically apply to stimulate and awaken the body's inner energies to have a life of their own within us. What are these energies and what might that life be?

To keep it simple, we often refer to the inner energies as being *neurobiological*, which indeed they are. In yoga terminology, the energies are called *prana* – on the move in this case. In tantra, the energy, once awakened, is recognized as sexual in origin – an expansion of essences from the vast storehouse of sexual energy in the pelvic region to permeate the entire body, and also radiate beyond the body into the environment as a non-physical essence. The tantric view may be the most useful in terms of understanding the symptoms that accompany an inner energy awakening. Very often, the sexual component is noticed experientially with advancement in yoga.

All of this also comes under the broad heading of *kundalini*, which is a well-known term nowadays, though still little understood. Whatever our terminology or understanding, clearly something profound is going on inside us energetically (or neurobiologically) as we undertake yoga practices.

Let's take a closer look at this phenomenon from the perspective of kundalini, which is the most ancient and well-developed body of knowledge on the ecstatic side of the human spiritual transformation equation.

Kundalini Primer

There are vast mythologies that have grown up around the inner workings of human spiritual transformation, incorporating various terminologies to describe this natural process. Whole religions have been spun from these mythologies, in the same way they have been for thousands of years in relation to natural events in the external environment. Here we will depart from myth (if not from terminology) and stick with the internal workings of the human nervous system, with the primary aim being to promote spiritual progress measured by our own experience.

The neurobiology of enlightenment is actually quite simple, though the journey itself is less so. We will try and keep both the journey and the mechanics of transformation as simple as possible. Indeed, without simplicity, there is little chance of success on this quest. It would be like trying to drive a car without the simplicity of operation supplied by a steering wheel, and with no view through the windshield to see where we are going!

Kundalini means *coiled serpent*, which means *latent or stored energy*. Once awakened, the term "kundalini" is still used, though in its dynamic mode it can hardly be regarded as being entirely latent anymore. The seat of this energy resides in our pelvic region, and is none other than the vast storehouse of our sexual energy. Under normal circumstances, the only demand made on this energy is for reproductive sexual activities, which is a primary purpose for it, of course – perpetuation of the species. However, it is well understood that, if sexual activity is minimized, a buildup of this energy occurs, and can overflow into creative behavior, athletic achievements, destructive behavior, or all of these. In other words, sexual energy has the potential to be expanded to other uses besides reproduction. In tantra, direct means can be applied to make good use of the principle of expanding the use of sexual energy, and this is fully covered elsewhere in the AYP writings.

It is also possible to promote the expansion of sexual energy to higher functioning in the nervous system by means that are less directly focused on sexuality, and this is where the mudras and bandhas come in.

Before we get into the specific methods, we should mention a bit about the neurobiology of kundalini.

First of all, there is a primary channel that kundalini takes up through the body as it evolves to higher manifestation within us. It is the central spinal nerve, also called the *sushumna* in yoga terminology. For our purposes, the spinal nerve is synonymous with the spinal cord in the center of the spinal column, and is the primary channel of awakening of kundalini in the body. It is the primary channel both in the flow of energy and in the experience of ecstatic conductivity that arises. The spinal nerve is also the foundation and link between the traditional energy plexus centers located in the nervous system, called *chakras*, as well as the tens of thousands of nerves fanning out to every part of our body.

So, kundalini begins in the pelvic region, awakens the spinal nerve, and from there reaches out through our nervous system to energize and illuminate every cell in our body. There are numerous biological functions involved in this overall process, many which can be directly observed as our spiritual progress advances. The mudras and bandhas are for stimulating these processes.

The end result of kundalini awakening, in conjunction with the cultivation of inner silence through deep meditation, is the enlightenment of the individual. It is a long term process, not one that occurs overnight, and this is why the building of an effective daily practice promoting these developments over time is, by far, the most important part of any system of yoga.

The next chapter provides more detail on the kundalini journey. Now let's look at the mudras and bandhas which play a vital role in the awakening and cultivation of ecstatic kundalini.

Instructions for Mudras and Bandhas

The human nervous system is a marvelous creation of nature, with capabilities that reach far beyond what is generally understood about it today, even by the most advanced sciences. The exception is the science of yoga, whose business is not only to understand the far-reaching capabilities of the human nervous system, but to accelerate the natural evolution of them. Taken all together, the practices of yoga are for that.

Mudras and bandhas have a special role to play in the grand scheme of the purification and opening of our nervous system to higher expression of our inherent divine qualities – peace, energy, creativity, compassion, and great happiness. However, it is important to understand that mudras and bandhas do not stand alone in this endeavor. In fact, if taken alone, mudras and bandhas amount to little more than weird exercises, and have been ridiculed as such by those who do not know their purpose. So let's first be clear that mudras and bandhas are only of benefit when combined in a routine of other yoga practices that provide the essential foundation for their effective use. These other yoga practices consist primarily of deep meditation and spinal breathing pranayama. There are others, but these two cover the basic prerequisites for mudras and bandhas – the cultivation of inner silence in meditation and the cultivation of the initial purification and opening in the spinal nerve through spinal breathing to facilitate the rise of ecstatic conductivity. Once these two practices are well established, then the use of mudras and bandhas can become a productive pursuit. So, let's be sure to start from that point in the development of our practice routine as we approach mudras and bandhas. If we don't, it will be like trying to build a castle in the air.

Mudra means *seal*, as in sealing a path or promoting a particular energy flow. Bandha means *lock*, as in blocking the flow of energy in a particular direction and thereby coaxing it in the opposite direction. Interestingly, most of the bandhas (blocks) have dynamic versions which are mudras (seals), or at least mudra-like in their performance and effects, hastening the flow of energy through particular neurobiological pathways. Sometimes there can be some confusion about whether a practice is a mudra, a bandha, or an asana, depending on how it is used, and when. We don't mind about that. Much better we should learn the practices themselves and make the best use of them.

On a practical level, mudras and bandhas can be either cause or effect in the overall scheme of yoga. This means that sometimes mudras would like to happen by themselves, by virtue of our purifying and opening nervous system. This does not mean we cast our fate to the four winds and pursue willy-nilly whatever may be cropping up in our yoga routine. It only means that we will receive clues from within on when the time may come to consider adding particular mudras or bandhas into our structured routine, or perhaps even to back off them if the stimulation is becoming too much. <u>All of yoga is a blending of the intentional with the instinctive – a balance of these two for optimal progress with safety.</u>

Most of the mudras and bandhas covered here are the ones associated with *cause* in spiritual practice. We know them as such because they act directly on the spinal nerve, or on neurobiology that is in close proximity to it. We will also discuss a few mudras that are more likely to be *effect* in spiritual practice, mainly associated with the hands, arms and torso.

At the end of the discussion on individual mudras and bandhas, we will tie it all together by covering the emergence of the *whole body mudra*, which is a marriage of the intentional with the instinctive aspects of the great tree of yoga. This is an expression of our own nervous system as it evolves to higher functioning. The whole body mudra is an effect of our yoga practice. Cause can yield effect, and effect can yield cause in many aspects of yoga practice. We call it the *interconnectedness* of the many aspects of yoga expressing naturally through our neurobiology.

As mentioned earlier, there is some overlap between asanas and mudras and bandhas. For this reason, we find two mudras (maha mudra and yoga mudra) and a bandha (abdominal lift/uddiyana) in the asana routine in the previous chapter. And we find an asana (siddhasana) included with mudras and bandhas here in this chapter, due to its being part of sitting practices rather than the asana routine.

Mulabandha (root lock)

The spinal nerve is the main highway in the body as far as inner energy awakening is concerned. It begins at the base of the spine in the region of the anus and perineum, and ends at the point between the eyebrows. Traditionally, the spinal nerve and all of its neurobiological connections are classified into three zones – lower, middle, and upper. These three zones are also called *knots* (granthis) when in an unpurified condition, with the practices of yoga being for the purpose of *untying* them. All of the mudras and bandhas are related to one or more of these zones, or knots, for the purpose of purifying and opening them, and for stimulating the flow of inner energy.

Mulabandha is the first of three primary bandhas that can be used in various ways within a yoga routine. It is also called the *root lock*. None of the three bandhas stand alone. Yet, we are taking them on one at a time here for the sake of clarity and a step-by-step building up of their use in an integrated way.

Stated most simply, mulabandha is a gentle squeezing of the anal sphincter muscle. Just an easy flex and hold. Along with that we do a gentle lift of the pelvic floor from the perineum up through the pelvic region. It begins in the anus and perineum (root), and reaches up through the pelvis. A slight contraction of the lower abdomen will occur with the lift up through the pelvis from the root.

Mulabandha can be held for as long as comfortable and then released. Then it can be initiated again as comfort allows. No doubt you are trying it now. That is fine. Just take it easy and don't overdo it. It takes some time to develop some comfort with this bandha. It will take a few weeks or months of regular practice to develop some familiarity.

Variations in anal sphincter activity during mulabandha can occur with breathing, particularly during spinal breathing pranayama, where our contractions and releases of the anal sphincter and pelvic floor may find a rhythm in relation to inhalation and exhalation. There is no best way to do this, but the tendency can arise during spinal breathing especially. The important thing is that mulabandha is occurring in a regular fashion, once we feel ready and have decided to do it. In the dynamic mode of flexing and releasing, mulabandha has another name, *asvini mudra,* which goes to show that the names can be as flexible as the practices. It is the cause and effect we are interested in.

You may notice some energy moving right away when beginning mulabandha. There might be some heat coming up, a flushed feeling, or even some sexual arousal. Any or all of these are normal. It may feel very awkward and mechanical – sort of clunky. This too is normal.

Keep in mind that we are doing something that we may have never done before with any sort of ongoing intention. So, naturally, it will be unfamiliar. Imagine what it would be like to begin writing with the opposite hand you usually write with. Would it be smooth and easy? Not likely. But, with time and practice it would become smooth and easy. It is the same with mulabandha, and all the mudras and bandhas. They start out pretty strange and awkward, and over time become graceful and ecstatic. The mudras and bandhas start out like ugly ducklings, and end up like beautiful swans. And so do we in our yoga practice.

Uddiyana Bandha (abdominal lock)

Let's continue up the body and look at the second primary bandha, called uddiyana bandha, or the *abdominal lock*. It is also called the *abdominal lift*, which is how it is named in the asana discussion in the previous chapter, where it is included as posture #11. Instructions for a standing version of it are provided there. To review, in practicing uddiyana we expel the air fully from our lungs and pull the abdomen inward by lifting the diaphragm upward into the lung cavity. This is held for several five-second durations, or longer, as comfortable.

Uddiyana means *to fly up*, which will become apparent to many as soon as the practice is used. The inner energy literally flies up!

There is a natural connection between mulabandha and uddiyana bandha, and they can be practiced together. Mulabandha stimulates the inner energy upward from the vast storehouse in the pelvic region, and uddiyana bandha hastens the energy higher through the midsection. While the primary channel for the energy flow is the spinal nerve, the effects can be felt throughout the body. When the main neurobiological channel is filled with the surging life force, all the subsidiary channels are immediately filled also, to the extent they can be according to the present degree of purification in the nervous system. No nerve or cell in the body is left untouched by the flow of energy in the spinal nerve.

There is an advanced version of uddiyana called *nauli*. It is dynamic, meaning it involves rhythmic movement, rather than holding a static position.

Nauli means *to churn*, and is accomplished by alternately flexing the left and right abdominal muscles to achieve a twirling effect. This is done in the same position as standing uddiyana, while flexing the abdominal muscles (like when doing a sit-up), first against one knee through the supporting arm, and then against the other knee through the other supporting arm (see illustration #11 in the previous chapter). This leads to the ability to control the flexing of left and right abdominal muscles separately, the key to accomplishing the twirling effect. Nauli is for stimulating the higher functioning of the digestive system.

Like uddiyana bandha, nauli is done with other mudras and bandhas, depending on the level of practice we have attained so far. Nauli is typically practiced during asanas at the same spot in the routine as uddiyana bandha, adding 10-20 twirls in each direction. Additional instructions on nauli can be found in the *AYP Easy Lessons* book. Nauli is a powerful enhancement and should not be attempted until the yoga routine of asanas and sitting practices are well established. And then it should be measured and self-paced with prudence for steady, safe progress. As with uddiyana bandha, a short duration of nauli practice will go a long way.

Jalandhara Bandha (chin lock)

The third primary bandha is jalandhara bandha, which means *chin lock*. It is performed by letting the chin go down toward the hollow of the throat to the degree it is comfortable. We don't force it. If the chin only goes halfway with comfort, this is good performance of the jalandhara bandha. It is like any other yoga practice in that respect. We go to our comfortable limit, and that is perfect performance of the practice for us at that time. Over weeks, months and years of regular practice, our limit may naturally extend, and that is how we gradually cultivate our practice. This is true of everything in yoga.

Jalandhara bandha is a two-directional practice, energy-wise. While inner energy naturally comes up from the pelvic region through the spinal nerve with good purifying and opening effects, it also naturally turns around when it reaches the head and comes back down the front by a different route which is oriented toward the gastrointestinal tract.

When we practice jalandhara bandha, we can feel the two-directional nature of it. When our spinal nerve becomes sufficiently sensitive, as we lower our chin, we can feel a tugging all the way through the nerve to the root. At the same time, we can feel the drawing down of energy from the head into the throat and chest cavity. So we are going in two directions with jalandhara bandha at the same time.

Keep in mind that we are talking about neurobiological energy moving through the nervous system, and as such, it has biochemical processes associated with it. While there will be an etheric quality to our experiences of inner energy flow, there are also underlying biological functions occurring throughout the body associated with human spiritual transformation. All of this goes through continuous refinement as our practices and experiences advance over time.

Jalandhara bandha is part of an important turning point in these neurobiological processes, from rising up the spinal nerve into the brain, to descending through the gastrointestinal system, where there is a recycling upward again, combined with the essences rising from the pelvic region. It is a complicated process, which becomes readily observable through inner sensations and visions as progress continues on the path of yoga.

As with mulabandha and uddiyana bandha, there is a dynamic version of jalandhara bandha, which greatly enhances the power of the practice. We call it *dynamic jalandhara* or *chin pump*.

Chin pump involves gently rotating the head in a circular motion in one direction with a gentle swoop toward the hollow of the throat on each forward down swing, with care being taken not to strain the neck. Then, after a predetermined duration (5 or 10 rotations), we reverse the direction of head rotation to go the other way. The chin pump can be practiced with a full breath retained (taking a new breath when reversing the direction of rotation), and with the other mudras and bandhas applied to create a very powerful practice producing much purification in the head, upper body, and beyond.

Please note: We do not start off our career in mudras and bandhas with the most powerful versions of these practices. To take them on, a stable routine of asanas and sitting practices is necessary. Then new practices can be incorporated step-by-step when we are ready, beginning with the basic versions. We have touched on some of the enhancements here to give an idea how practices can evolve over time. More detail on integrating the mudras and bandhas into the daily practice routine will be covered further on in this book. Also, additional study on advanced practices covered in *AYP Easy Lessons* book is suggested.

Sambhavi Mudra (third eye seal)

There is a remarkable connection between the brain and the neurobiological refinements that occur throughout the body in connection with the processes of human spiritual transformation. Jalandhara stimulates this connection, as do uddiyana, and mulabandha, lower down. When awakened, the spinal nerve becomes a continuum of ecstatic sensitivity between the brain and the root (perineum/anus), and to all parts of the nervous system, both near and far from the central channel.

Sambhavi mudra is a physical maneuver involving the eyes and brow that brings both stimulation and control to the process of whole body ecstatic awakening. Sambhavi mudra is a gentle raising of the eyes toward the point between the eyebrows, and an equally gentle intention to furrow the center of the brow. The eyes lift up a bit along with an intention to bring the two eyebrows together. That's it. Nothing too dramatic or extreme.

Before the spinal nerve has been ecstatically awakened, sambhavi mudra may not feel like much. In fact, it may seem awkward and clumsy. Most of the mudras and bandhas do when tried for the first time. With time, they become familiar and comfortable. And once the spinal nerve begins to awaken ecstatically, well, the mudras and bandhas become highly pleasurable. This is especially true of sambhavi mudra. Why? Because it acts directly on the *third eye*.

The so-called *third eye* is the area of the brain that extends from the center brow back to the center of the head and then down into the spine via the medulla oblongata (brain stem). This area in the brain encompasses a specialized neurology, and the pituitary and pineal glands, which together are capable of producing profound effects throughout the entire nervous system, once the connections are stimulated and awakened. The mudras and bandhas provide this stimulation in the three zones mentioned previously – lower, middle and upper.

Sambhavi focuses on the third eye, which is called *ajna* in yogic terminology. Interestingly, ajna means *command*. Once the ecstatic awakening occurs in the spinal nerve the reason becomes clear enough. The steady expansion of ecstatic energy flow throughout the body is stimulated and regulated by the ajna through the mudras that directly access that part of the neurobiology in the head, with sambhavi being a primary one.

The awakening of ecstatic energy in the spinal nerve opens us to the vast reaches of inner space, and many the blessings that come with that. Sambhavi and all of the mudras and bandhas have a key role to play in this. As we become familiar with the mudras and bandhas, and learn to combine them with our core practices, we find ourselves in a good position to solve the entire puzzle of human spiritual transformation.

Siddhasana (perfect pose or seat)

Now we will go back to the bottom of the spinal nerve again. While, technically, siddhasana is an asana, it fits right in with the mudras and bandhas, particularly as we look toward assembling them into a usable routine of twice-daily practices that can be engaged in over the long term with ease and good results.

We did not sign up here to retreat into a cave to engage in all of these practices from dawn until dusk. Most of us have to work for a living, raise a family, and be active in the world. So we need to do our spiritual practices in a compact routine that fits into our busy day, and in such a way so our normal daily activities will naturally advance our inner growth.

We have spoken about asanas (postures) and how they can be used to prepare us for sitting practices such as spinal breathing pranayama and deep meditation. We will soon learn how to incorporate the mudras and bandhas into our sitting practices in a way that is easy and takes little to no extra time. Efficiency!

Siddhasana is a practice like that – it is something we can do while we are doing our spinal breathing pranayama, and also during our deep meditation, once we have become comfortable in it.

Siddhasana means *perfect pose*. Sometimes it is called the *seat of the perfected ones*. But let's not be too presumptuous. Let's just call it a good way to sit in our pranayama and meditation practice.

Why?

One simple reason – siddhasana provides a gentle stimulation of the energy in our pelvic region. Siddhasana is performed by sitting with one of our heels underneath us and pressed on the perineum – the area between the genitals and the anus. It does not matter which heel. It can be alternated if need be. And if the heel can't reach, we can use a suitable substitute object, like a rubber ball or rolled up sock, to accomplish the same function. We will not stand on ceremony. There is no such thing as perfection in any of these practices. Only effective, or not so effective. We will take effective, thank you very much.

The idea in siddhasana, the essential principle, is to have some pressure at the perineum while we are sitting. The best time to learn the habit of siddhasana is during our spinal breathing pranayama. That is five or ten minutes in the seat. Once we gain the habit and become comfortable in siddhasana, then we can do it in meditation too, which means a half-hour or more in the seat. This is very good for ecstatically awakening the spinal nerve, and the entire body.

If we are accustomed to sitting with legs crossed in our pranayama and meditation, then siddhasana will be a short step forward. It is suggested to do it sitting on a soft surface, like a bed, with back support. Then we will have good control of how much pressure is placed on the perineum by the heel. It should not be excessive pressure, not to the degree of cutting off circulation to the genitals, especially in the case of the male. If the heel is properly placed under and behind the pubic bone, blood circulation will not be an issue.

Here is a sketch showing the easy performance of siddhasana:

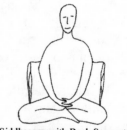

Siddhasana with Back Support

If we do not sit with crossed legs during our pranayama and meditation, the same effect can be achieved while sitting in a chair with a suitable object placed underneath the perineum.

One might ask about the so-called *lotus posture* (padmasana), which is performed by tying the legs in a pretzel-like knot, with both feet up on the opposite thighs. It is a posture that is familiar to many, if not performed by many. It has its benefits for advanced practitioners, but does not perform the same function as siddhasana – stimulation at the perineum. Plus, siddhasana is much easier to do, and can be simulated with a suitable object substituting for the heel at the perineum. So, for our purposes, we will stay with siddhasana.

Kechari Mudra (seal of inner space)
　　Somewhere along the path of yoga, most of us will experience a natural reflex of the tongue being drawn up to the roof of the mouth and back. It happens when the inner energies begin to move. In fact, all of the mudras and bandhas are naturally stimulated in this way, which makes for some interesting possibilities. More on that later.
　　The drawing up and back of the tongue is called kechari mudra. Kechari means to *fly through inner space*. What does this mean? Only that, with the initial rise of ecstatic conductivity, our inner dimensions begin to become available to us experientially, and the tongue drawing up and back accentuates this phenomenon. It is a natural development in our neurobiology.
　　What may be surprising about kechari is how far the tongue can go in this direction, particularly if given some help. We will talk about two stages of development here:

Stage 1 – The tip of the tongue reaching the point on the roof of the mouth where the hard and soft palates meet.

Stage 2 – The tip of the tongue reaching behind the soft palate, and the tongue going up into the nasal pharynx cavity to find the spiritually erogenous edge of the nasal septum, located directly above the place where the hard and soft palates meet on the roof of the mouth.

The two stages of kechari mudra are illustrated in the following diagrams:

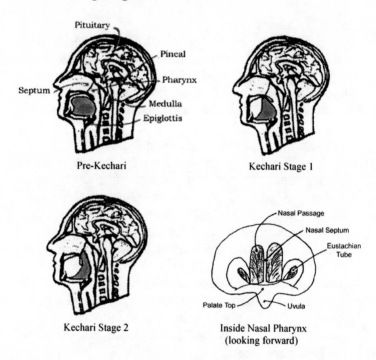

Pre-Kechari

Kechari Stage 1

Kechari Stage 2

Inside Nasal Pharynx
(looking forward)

For additional stages of kechari mudra, see the *AYP Easy Lessons* book.

Stage 2 kechari is accomplished by pushing the tongue forward, once the tip has gotten behind the edge of the soft palate – entry may be achieved on the left side, right side, or in the center. Upon entry, when the tongue is pushed forward, the soft palate opens downward like a trap door, and the tongue easily goes forward to find the nasal septum. In the beginning, a finger pressing the tongue back from underneath can aid in getting behind the soft palate. Later on, stage 2 can be entered with no finger help. Nasal breathing is not blocked in stage 2 kechari.

In both of these stages of kechari the nerves in the nasal septum are being stimulated – in stage 1 from underneath through the roof of the mouth, and in stage 2 by direct contact of the tongue with the edge of the nasal septum. These nerves can also be stimulated indirectly by contact with the tongue in other areas in the mouth and throughout the soft palate. Kechari mudra also acts on the neurobiology in the throat, which is related to the effects created in jalandhara bandha.

At this point in time, we may or may not feel inclined to intentionally pull the tongue up and back into kechari mudra. However, after months or years of daily deep meditation, spinal breathing pranayama, and the other mudras and bandhas, the tendency will tend to increase for kechari mudra to occur on its own. Energetically it will happen. Effective yoga practices will sooner or later lead to kechari mudra, just as puberty leads eventually to a maturing of sexual function. Kechari is one of the tell-tale signs of a second kind of puberty going on in the body – *spiritual puberty*. Once the kechari urge arrives, we may feel inclined to help it along. This is the natural way to approach kechari, without forcing it by will. This is preferred, especially in considering stage 2.

Physically, the primary inhibitor of kechari mudra is the membrane under the tongue, called the *frenulum* or *frenum*. In yoga, the frenum is regarded as a hymen – a restricting tissue to be penetrated when a strong urge to enter kechari mudra has arrived. This is the energetic reflex which has been mentioned.

Once the urge has arrived, the tongue will go up and back. Then it becomes a matter of what to do about the frenum. A small number of people are born with little or no frenum under the tongue and are able to perform kechari stages 1 and 2 with little or no effort. This may or may not be an advantage, depending on the person's spiritual condition, and what other yoga practices they have been doing. Being born with no frenum under the tongue is not a guarantee of spiritual acumen. Without a spiritual inclination and a full range of practices occurring, kechari stage 2 may be little more than a parlor trick, producing the illusion of swallowing the tongue as it disappears behind the soft palate. It is not swallowing the tongue – only hiding the tongue behind the soft palate in the cavity of the nasal pharynx, which is above the mouth. On the other hand, for those who are yogically inclined, being born with little or no frenum can be a gift, enabling easy entry into kechari mudra. For the rest of us, some work is necessary.

In the ancient *Hatha Yoga Pradipika*, trimming of the frenum is prescribed using a sharp blade, taking cuts the size of a hair, with healing in-between. These days we have the advantages of technology. Small sterilized cuticle nippers (like small wire cutter pliers) can be used with greater precision and more safety to take tiny snips the size of a hair on the stretched edge of the frenum in the center, with days or weeks to heal in-between snips. With such an approach, properly executed, little to no blood will be drawn. It is reasonably safe and will lead to success in due course.

Some practitioners who are in a hurry to enter stage 2 kechari may seek a doctor to reduce the frenum surgically. It is a matter of personal preference. We can only say that the urge toward kechari will increase naturally once our nervous system has been sufficiently purified and opened by our other yoga practices. Then the means for dealing with the frenum will be according to individual preference. Or, perhaps the frenum, as is, will not restrict progress into kechari mudra at all. We will find out when the time comes.

More detail on trimming the frenum under the tongue for entering higher stages of kechari mudra can be found in *AYP Easy Lessons* book, and in the *AYP online support forums*. Information on both resources can be found on the last page of this book.

Yoni Mudra (spinal nerve seal)

Now we will begin tying the mudras together, integrating the effects in the lower, middle and upper body. Yoni mudra does that, while adding several new elements of practice as well.

So far, we have been discussing pieces of the puzzle – mulabandha, uddiyana bandha, jalandhara bandha, sambhavi mudra, siddhasana and kechari mudra. In yoni mudra, we put all of these together, and add breath retention (kumbhaka) and additional gentle stimulation of the eyes with the index fingers. Traditionally, yoni mudra involves closing all the orifices of the head using all ten fingers, but here we will use an abbreviated version that is much easier to do, and very effective.

We begin by sitting in siddhasana, to whatever degree we are practicing that at present. If we have not begun to use siddhasana, or other mudras and bandhas already discussed, we can still do yoni mudra while leaving those out. But for greatest effectiveness it will be good to have some familiarity with all of the practices covered so far. In fact, for ideal results with any mudra, it is best if there is a regular routine in place using spinal breathing pranayama and deep meditation as the foundation.

So, to practice yoni mudra, we sit in siddhasana with back support and inhale slowly and steadily up the spine from the root to the brow. Once we have a full breath, we hold it.

Then, with eyes closed, we take the tips of our index fingers (the first finger after the thumb) and rest them under the eyeballs on top of the bone near the outside corners of our eye sockets. This will produce a gentle pressure on the eyes upward and centered toward the point between the eyebrows. The fingernails may have to be trimmed for this procedure to work properly. We do not force the eyes. Only exert a very gentle nudge from the lower outside corners of the eyes toward the point between the eyebrows. The elbows can hang down comfortably near our torso. It is not necessary to hold the arms up in the air. While we are doing this maneuver with the eyes, we also include a gentle intention to furrow the center brow, just as we do in sambhavi mudra.

At the same time we are nudging the eyes with our index fingers while having the gentle intention to furrow the brow, we close the outside nostrils of our nose with the middle fingers (the finger between the index finger and ring finger), still retaining the air we have just inhaled. We keep our mouth closed, and let the gentle pressure of our retained breath go into our nasal passages from the inside.

Finally, at the same time, we perform mulabandha, uddiyana bandha, jalandhara bandha, sambhavi mudra and kechari mudra, each to the extent we are familiar and comfortable. It is a lot to do at once, but all of these elements are static, so once they are in place, they can be easily held. And this is how we stay until we are ready to exhale.

We do not strain with our breath retention. It is not a contest to see how long we can hold our breath. In fact, there is little benefit to extending breath retention beyond a comfortable limit. That may be only ten seconds for us, or twenty seconds, or maybe half a minute or more. We don't have to time it. We just hold the breath in until the urge to let it go comes, and then we let go by releasing the fingers on the nose and let the breath come out while tracing the spinal nerve back down from the center brow to the root. As we let the air out, we can relax all the mudras and bandhas we are doing. That is one cycle of yoni mudra.

Maha Mudra (great seal)

As discussed previously, a good start to our overall yoga routine of postures, pranayama and meditation is an easy set of asanas, and we have presented a series of postures in the previous chapter for that purpose. This is a basic set of asanas that can be also learned (with variations) at any yoga studio anywhere in the world. Two of the postures in this set of asanas have the name "mudra." Though basic instructions to perform them have already been given in the *Asana Starter Kit*, we will talk about them some more here from the standpoint of mudra application.

Maha mudra (great seal) is a posture that is sometimes used as a jumping off point from basic yoga asanas into more serious pursuit of advanced yoga practices and experiences. With maha mudra, we take a decidedly more direct focus on purifying and opening the spinal nerve during the head to knee pose (posture #4 in the previous chapter) by adding physical pressure at the perineum, breath retention, and other mudras and bandhas discussed above, much in the way we have done with yoni mudra.

To supercharge the basic head to knee posture, we come up on the heel to increase pressure at the perineum as in siddhasana, and we inhale before leaning over and hold the breath inside (kumbhaka) as we lean over. At the same time we perform mulabandha, uddiyana bandha, jalandhara bandha, sambhavi mudra, and kechari mudra while we hold the posture at our comfortable limit.

Maha mudra can be performed as part of our regular asana routine, with as few or as many of the extra components desired, depending on the level of proficiency we have attained with the mudras and bandhas, and the status of our inner energies. We do not wish to overdo. In its most basic form, maha mudra is a simple sitting head to one knee stretch, with nothing else added. You can take it from there according to your inclination and level of practice. Be sure to keep maha mudra contained within a reasonable time duration in relation to the rest of the asana routine. The basic posture duration is 10 seconds by inward count – one, two, three, four, etc... If 20 seconds is used for each posture in the routine, including for maha mudra, then this is getting to be a pretty hefty asana routine, and keep an eye out for excessive energy flows during or after the routine.

Keep in mind that, very often, symptoms of overdoing can come with a delayed effect, sometimes much later. Always pay attention to resulting experiences as you weave these powerful practices into your routine one at a time. This is especially true of mudras and bandhas that are supplemented with breath retention (kumbhaka).

Breath retention greatly increases the tendency of the inner ecstatic energies to awaken. When a slight deficit of oxygen is created in the body in a systematic way, the life force in the pelvic region moves to compensate. Breath retention in conjunction with mudras and bandhas should be prudently self-paced to avoid excessive energy flow in the body.

Yoga Mudra (seal of yoga)

Yoga mudra (seal of yoga) is also found in the set of asanas covered in the previous chapter, and taught in most yoga studios around the world. As described and shown as posture #7, yoga mudra is sitting with legs crossed and leaning forward as far as comfortable. It is a natural stretching of the spinal nerve, with stimulation on the lower end and inversion on the upper end. Because of its simplicity, yoga mudra is one of the most common automatic yogas that can occur during sitting practices. It is experienced as an urge to let the torso come forward and down as we are sitting in spinal breathing pranayama or deep meditation. So, while we are doing yoga mudra as a regular part of our asanas, it can also appear during our sitting practices without our even thinking about it. In that case, we just gently favor the practice we are doing. If the torso has to come down for a time, we can let it. We don't have to fight against it. But neither do we favor it over the practice we are doing. If the torso comes down, after a little while, we can come back up into the sitting practice we are doing. Very easy, like that.

Automatic Yoga and the Hand Mudras

During spinal breathing pranayama and deep meditation, as the inner energies begin to move, sometimes the body tends to move also, as though animated from within. The whole upper body may tend to sway, or move into asana-like postures, even as we are sitting quietly on our meditation seat.

Along with the swaying, some arm movements can happen, as though a dance is occurring. Indeed, the inner energy flows that are natural to all human beings have influenced dance in many cultures, whether within the spiritual traditions, or outside them.

An effective way to seal the flow of inner energies in the hands, arms and upper body, is to engage the *hand mudras*. These come in several varieties (chin or jnana), which involve completing an energy circuit between the thumb and first finger. During pranayama and meditation this can be done with the hands resting on the thighs or knees, with the palms facing either down or up. The result will be a smoother flow of the energy in the arms and upper body, and a tendency toward less physical movement. In other words, more efficient flow of ecstatic energy.

In our approach here, we do not regard the hand mudras as a primary cause of spiritual progress, but as an effect coming from the awakening of ecstatic energy in the upper body, and the arms in particular. When this happens, an energy circuit being closed is easily noticed when the thumb and first finger are joined. Before this, the hand mudras are only gestures having little to do with inner development. And, of course, this is how we normally see them, as gestures in the stereotype pose of the yogi sitting like a pretzel on a rock with hand mudras firmly established on knees. We do not seek that sort of imagery here – only to promote the process of human spiritual transformation by the most efficient means possible.

The suggestion is to engage in the core practices of spinal breathing pranayama and deep meditation. If the inclination is there to do asanas, then do those beforehand. With all of that, the call to mudras and bandhas will be felt coming from within. When we feel called to hand mudras, we will know we have some inner energy awakening occurring. Another small step on our long journey to enlightenment.

Whole Body Mudra

So far, we have discussed a pretty long list of mudras and bandhas, covering basic practices and enhancements. We have mentioned that these are the components of a big puzzle, which, when put together, will promote overall ecstatic awakening in our nervous system.

At first glance, the means seem complicated. But it is not really as complicated as it appears, because there is only one nervous system – ours – and all of these means are automatically interconnected within us.

We will know that this is true as our inner energies begin to awaken. Then, all of the mudras and bandhas we have been talking about begin to operate as a single coordinated function just like the complex biological functions that are occurring within us right now sustaining our physical existence. We are just cultivating another level of automatic functioning – a very special one associated with spiritual transformation.

When ecstatic conductivity first begins to stir, we may notice a connection between our head and our root, a sensation and flexing at our root when we raise our eyes. That is a connection between sambhavi and mulabandha. Then it will expand to more of the mudras and bandhas. In time, all of the mudras and bandhas become connected. If we are doing mudras and bandhas as part of our regular daily practice routine, this promotes the development of rising inner connectivity and ecstatic conductivity. It all works together like that.

There is no one *magic bullet* in yoga – there are many interconnected means that gradually merge to become a single evolutionary process incorporating a wide range of neurobiological processes within us. This is especially true of the mudras and bandhas, which depend on each other and the rest of our yoga practices to be effective.

Then, when the eyes move devotionally, all the mudras will subtly move by automatic ecstatic reflex. Ahhh... That is why we nudge these mudras along in our practice routine until ecstatic conductivity comes up. We are building the habits, setting up for further evolution in the nervous system. Then, with ecstatic conductivity on the rise, there is only one mudra – the whole body mudra made up of all the parts.

Sambhavi mudra is the leader of it. That's why we see pictures of the sages with their eyes raised. They are in whole body ecstatic bliss just from eyes raised, with the whole body mudra activated and divine energy radiating out in all directions. This divine ecstatic reflex will be with us 24 hours per day.

Filling in the Practice Routine

As mentioned, mudras and bandhas do not constitute a practice routine by themselves, even when combined together in the large scope mudras like yoni mudra and maha mudra. Yoni mudra and maha mudra, for all their wonderful effects, are but part of the overall practice routine – important cogs in the wheel of yoga. How do we go about building the mudras and bandhas into our yoga practice so we can steadily cultivate the desired effects over time? How do we stitch this all together into something that will be practical, effective and safe?

In these busy times, we are fortunate to be able to add most of the mudras and bandhas into our existing practice routine without adding more time. This is very good news! Mudras and bandhas are physical habits we would like to cultivate. Once they become automatic habits, mudras and bandhas tend to take on a life of their own in response to the inner energies they are awakening. But how do we develop these mudra and bandha habits without disrupting our daily practices? Doing them for 10 seconds here and there in our asana routine will not be enough to form a solid habit. And we do not wish to be disrupting deep meditation by diverting attention to physical maneuvers. That won't work.

It turns out that our spinal breathing pranayama session is an ideal time to be cultivating the mudras and bandhas. Therefore, the first thing we need before undertaking mudras and bandhas, is a stable routine of spinal breathing pranayama, preferably with a deep meditation session right after it. Detailed instructions for these core practices can be found in the *AYP Easy Lessons* book, and in the concise *AYP Enlightenment Series* books.

Add-ons to Spinal Breathing Pranayama Session

Once we have the foundation of a sitting practices routine, then we are in the best position to be cultivating the mudras and bandhas, beyond those we may be doing for short periods of time in our asana routine. Sitting practices, and spinal breathing pranayama in particular, provide much more time for mudras and bandhas. If we are doing spinal breathing pranayama for five or ten minutes, then that is five or ten minutes we can be developing the habits of mudras and bandhas, without adding any time to our practice routine. So, how do we proceed? One step at a time…

Once we are stable in spinal breathing pranayama, followed by deep meditation, we can consider adding mudras and bandhas. If we are starting from the beginning, we are talking about several months before starting mudras and bandhas, at least. Once we do begin mudras and bandhas, we do not take them on all at once. We can't expect to achieve success with an "all at once" approach to yoga practices, any more than we can expect to be successful in driving a car at high speed the first time we get in it. It takes time to develop the skills and familiarity necessary to effectively and safely drive the car. It is like that with yoga practices too. So we take a phased approach over time to ensure best results.

Let's assume we have done our prerequisite work for a few months (or many months), and now have a five-minute spinal breathing pranayama session followed by 20 minutes of deep meditation, forming a foundation for beginning mudras and bandhas during sitting practices. There are two practices we can add once we feel stable in spinal breathing – mulabandha and sambhavi mudra. Recall that mulabandha is a gentle compression of the anal sphincter muscle accompanied by a slight lifting of the pelvic floor, and that sambhavi mudra is a gentle raising of the eyes accompanied by a gentle intention to furrow the center brow.

After a period of weeks or months, however long it takes to achieve good stability in our daily practice routine with mulabandha and sambhavi, additional elements can be added, with siddhasana (applying pressure at the perineum while sitting) being a good next step. Siddhasana can take months to stabilize, and it is suggested not to add anything else until it becomes second nature. In fact, it may be necessary to back off practices from time to time if excess energy is experienced. This backing off is called *self-pacing*, and is an essential part of building and maintaining our yoga practice routine. Everyone is different in terms of the matrix of inner obstructions being dissolved during yoga practices, and how that will be experienced, so the rate at which practices can be comfortably added and the course of self-pacing will be unique for each person.

It is very important that we develop the ability to back off when things are going too fast. It can mean that we add mulabandha during our full spinal breathing pranayama session today, and back off it tomorrow for a day or two. Then we can come back to it again when we feel ready. Likewise with sambhavi, siddhasana and the rest of the practices we are building into our routine. It goes like that – add a practice, stabilize it, which can mean backing off and restoring as we acclimate to the new levels of energy flowing inside, and then go on to adding the next practice. In this way, it can take many months, or even years, to develop our overall routine of practices, with mudras and bandhas being an important part – the golden threads in the tapestry of our yoga routine that help us awaken ecstatic conductivity.

With this approach, we are able to build our routine of practices at our own pace, and are not obliged to hang around waiting according to someone else's timetable. If we feel ready to move ahead, we can. But we'd better pace ourselves wisely each step along the way to avoid overdoing. As with most things, the freedom to act is accompanied by the responsibility to act wisely.

What we have found with thousands of practitioners using the AYP methods is that, with a little experience, nearly everyone is able to self-pace their practices with reasonable effectiveness. And so we keep moving ahead.

Once spinal breathing pranayama has become stable in our twice-daily routine, with mulabandha, sambhavi and siddhasana added, then we are in a position to consider kechari mudra. It starts as a simple lifting of the tongue to the palate during spinal breathing pranayama. Over time, kechari will evolve naturally, and will require self-pacing also – backing off as necessary from time to time to avoid excess energy flows.

Returning to the car driving analogy – we slow down when we come to a sharp curve or potholes in the road, and we speed up when we are on the smooth straightaway again. In this same way, we can gradually build up our yoga practice routine to achieve good progress with comfort and safety over the long haul.

Mudras and Bandhas as Stand-Alone Practice

Some of the mudras and bandhas can be done in stand-alone mode within our overall practice routine. Maha mudra and yoga mudra are individual mudras that are performed as part of the sequence of postures in our asana routine.

In sitting practices, yoni mudra and/or dynamic jalandhara (chin pump) can be performed as individual practices between spinal breathing pranayama and deep meditation. These should not be added to the routine at the same time. If our spinal breathing pranayama session is stable with the additions discussed already, then yoni mudra can be considered to add between spinal breathing and deep meditation. This would consist of only a few breath retentions (kumbhakas) starting out, and then going straight into deep meditation. Recall that yoni mudra includes the maneuvers of the fingers with the eyes and nose, plus slightly furrowed brow, during inward breath retention with mulabandha, uddiyana bandha, jalandhara bandha, plus sambhavi and kechari mudras, all to the degree we are comfortable. Three breath retentions will take only a few minutes, and then we are on to deep meditation, so yoni mudra adds only a few minutes to our practice routine.

The same goes for dynamic jalandhara (chin pump) which can be placed right after spinal breathing and yoni mudra, once we are stable in all previous practices undertaken. Like yoni mudra, chin pump should be limited to a few cycles of head rotation in each direction, with or without breath retention added, so will only take a few minutes also. If chin pump is added, yoni mudra can be moved to be after deep meditation (and samyama, if doing) and before the rest period at the end of our routine.

Mudras & Bandhas in Deep Meditation & Samyama

Deep meditation and samyama (the tri-limbed yoga practice introduced in Chapter 2) are different from spinal breathing pranayama, in that they require attention to be free to follow the procedures of practice. We do not use our deep meditation and samyama sessions (typically 20 minutes for meditation and 10 minutes for samyama) for developing mudras and bandhas, as this would distract us from the specific mental procedures being utilized. Once our mudras and bandhas have become automatic habits, developed largely during spinal breathing pranayama, then we may find them cropping up in our deep meditation and samyama sessions. This is fine, as long as we give them no attention other than what may occur normally during the procedures of these practices. In deep meditation, this means easily and comfortably coming back to our *mantra* whenever we realize we have drifted off from it. In samyama, it means continuing with the specific procedure of picking up and releasing our *sutras* in inner silence. See the *AYP Easy Lessons* book and other AYP writings for instructions on samyama.

The mudras and bandhas can be there during these mental procedures or not, and we do not mind them if they are. In this way, as we develop the habits of mudras and bandhas in spinal breathing, the automatic physical maneuvers may occur (usually subtly) during deep meditation and samyama, or at other times, including during our daily activity. And if they do not, that is okay too.

Over time, mudras and bandhas become a natural response in our body, both stimulating and responding to the flow of ecstatic energy within us.

The Overall Practice Routine

To help clarify how the mudras and bandhas are woven into an overall practice routine, consider the following. A routine like this can be undertaken twice-daily, before the morning and evening meal:

- During Asanas (10 min) – May include maha mudra, yoga mudra, and uddiyana bandha.

- During Spinal Breathing Pranayama (5-10 min) – May include mulabandha, sambhavi mudra, siddhasana, and kechari mudra.

- Yoni Mudra or Dynamic Jalandhara/chin pump (a few minutes) – May be undertaken as a stand-alone practice.

- During Deep Meditation (20 min) and Samyama (10 min) – Mudras and bandhas are not to be undertaken deliberately. They may occur as automatic habits. Siddhasana may be added when it can be performed without excessive distraction.

- Yoni Mudra (a few minutes) – May be included here as a stand-alone practice, if doing chin pump after spinal breathing pranayama.

- During Rest (5-10 min, corpse pose optional) – No deliberate practice of mudras and bandhas, though they may occur automatically.

As mentioned, mudras and bandhas might also occur automatically at any time during our regular daily activity. They can be quite subtle, natural and pleasant, as we have covered in discussing the *whole body mudra* earlier. This is an evolution of our inner neurobiology as we advance along the path of yoga and is a result of the combined effects of all of our practice. No one practice, or class of practices, will facilitate the entire result. An integration of practices is necessary.

If all this sounds complicated, it really is not, as long as we take things one step at a time, and continue with persistence and self-pacing over the long haul. Rome was not built in a day.

Keep in mind that in all of yoga we are purifying and opening the spinal nerve and, automatically through it, the entire nervous system. We have global techniques for this in the form of spinal breathing pranayama, deep meditation and samyama. And we have more targeted methods in the form of asanas, mudras and bandhas. In the case of targeted methods, we can think of the body being divided into three regions – lower, middle and upper – with techniques designed for each. As the regions become purified and opened, they dissolve to become whole body spiritual awakening.

The Rise of Inner Energy

There are two sides to the enlightenment equation, both occurring within our nervous system – the cultivation of inner silence, primarily through deep meditation and samyama, and the cultivation of ecstatic conductivity, primarily through pranayama, asanas, mudras, bandhas and tantric sexual methods.

No one magic bullet … rather, a full range of methods.

As inner silence and ecstatic conductivity come up within us, a blending of these two qualities occurs. This can be described as either a stilling of ecstatic energy, or an enlivening of inner silence. It is both. It can also be called the rise of *stillness in action*, which means that we become a channel of the divine flow from within. We come to know it as an outpouring of divine love.

Asanas, mudras and bandhas, are for aiding the ecstatic side of the equation, or the awakening of inner energy. How will we know that mudras and bandhas are working?

Simple. Sooner or later we will feel the movement of energy within us. Depending on our progress with a range of daily practices over months or years, we may or may not notice immediate results with mudras and bandhas. Everyone has a different matrix of inner obstructions to be cleared over time. Even when we notice inner energy moving, we will still have a long way to go with inner purification. The initial rise of inner energy can be felt in many possible ways. It can be felt as some pressure somewhere, which eventually gives way to a sensation that can be quite pleasurable. Or it may be pleasurable first, with other experiences coming up later. Any sequence of experiences is possible, depending on the course of our inner purification.

If we are doing a mudra or bandha in one location, we may feel a sensation in an entirely different location – a sure sign of energy conductivity occurring across the nervous system. Once it starts, it will keep developing over months and years. Eventually, we will know that all we see in this life is moving ecstatic silence. We will be the agent of that in our own experience, and as an automatic catalyst for the same evolutionary experience rising in everyone we encounter. Such is the nature of outpouring divine love.

Chapter 4 – Awakening Ecstatic Kundalini

Since ancient times, it has been known that human spiritual experience includes two components, one that brings great inner peace and forbearance, and another that brings great inner energy, ecstasy, and creative power. The latter has been called the *Holy Spirit* in the West, and *Kundalini* in the East. It has other names in the many cultures, religions and sects around the world. This inner energy is sometimes associated with *serpents* (recall that kundalini means *coiled serpent*), due to the sensations of undulating motion it can produce rising in and around the spinal column. Sometimes sensations of heat are also present, and the term *serpent fire* has been used to describe this. By whatever name, it is the same vast neurobiological potential residing within each of us. Whether dormant or awakened, kundalini is part of our internal functioning – our evolutionary birthright.

Though many have heard of kundalini, little is understood about it – especially the practical aspects of awakening this great resource within us in a progressive and safe manner. The annals of modern spiritual literature are filled with horror stories about spontaneous and/or premature kundalini awakenings, which can compromise physical and mental health. That is what happens when 1,000 watts of power is forced through a 100-watt light bulb. That 100-watt bulb needs quite a lot of conditioning before it can become a 1000-watt bulb.

Why does the imbalance happen? It has been due mainly to a lack of education both in the present, and in the past when the seeds of current energy upheavals have been planted. Indeed, a few people are born with energy imbalances, sometimes accompanied by strong spiritual aspirations – suggesting possible aggressive and unbalanced spiritual endeavors before this lifetime.

The good news is that there are effective ways to manage the unfoldment of kundalini, including help for those who may be having difficulty due to possible excessive inner energy endeavors in the past.

This is the scientific age, and there is no doubt that we can learn the correct applications of cause and effect in our yoga practices and our lifestyle to achieve good spiritual progress, while maintaining balance and safety. Why not? Humanity has done it with many powerful technologies, which are now used to great advantage, and with reasonable safety.

The same can be accomplished with the huge spiritual power that resides within each of us. The evolution of yoga to become a viable *applied science* offers rewards far beyond what we have imagined our ultimate capabilities to be. It is only a matter of developing the practical methodologies of cause and effect in an open source way, so the knowledge can be tested, refined and disseminated by many people on all sides. This is the way of applied science.

Asanas, mudras and bandhas have a key role to play in this evolution. The prudent application of these as part of an integrated twice-daily routine of yoga practices, with good application of the principles of *self-pacing*, can accelerate our spiritual evolution tremendously. At the same time, comfort and safety can be maintained so we can carry on our normal life at work, and at home with our family.

It is possible to have a realistic approach to awakening and accommodating the creative power of ecstatic kundalini in our life, while gaining the many practical benefits. It is only a matter of knowing how.

Symptoms and Remedies

When the inner energies begin to move in us as a result of yoga practices, there will be signs and symptoms of kundalini awakening. If the symptoms become excessive, there are a variety of means available to manage the process of awakening to provide for good progress with comfort and safety.

For many, just knowing that these symptoms are normal signs of ecstatic inner awakening can bring comfort to the process. Knowledge can go a long way toward relieving the concerns that can come with an inner awakening. No one is alone on this journey.

Symptoms

The symptoms of kundalini awakening are wide-ranging, and can include any combination of:

- Pleasurable or erotic sensations coming up the spine from the root (perineum/anus) to the head, or localized anywhere in-between. These sensations can be associated with the perception of a tiny silver thread in the spine in the early stages, to a large swirling multi-colored column of energy in later stages, encompassing the spine, the whole body and beyond.

- Pressure or aching in the head, or other areas where inner energy is encountering obstructions to smooth ecstatic flow.

- Radiating and/or undulating hot or cold currents in the body, localized or everywhere. The feelings can be both hot and cold at the same time, giving a radiant sensation like liniment, menthol or mint.

- Sweet flavors or aromas coming down from the nasal passages and pharynx into the mouth and throat.

- Sensations of insects crawling on the limbs, sometimes including pinches, pricking sensations, goosebumps or hair standing on end. In some cases, skin eruptions or rash can occur. The experience can also come in the form of itchy or erotic sensations in the feet and hands.

- Physical or electric-like jolts and jerks in the body. A tendency for automatic movements of head, torso and arms. In some cases, movement of objects or other unusual occurrences in the external environment may happen.

- Sudden inhalation or exhalation, or a rapid sequence of both, sometimes accompanied by vocalizations.

- Sounds inside – humming, buzzing, chimes, whistling, voices and other inner sounds. The head and heart spaces are prime areas for these.

- Visions – lights, shapes, landscapes and beings. Any of the senses can be involved.

- Strong emotions – ranging from extreme euphoria to the following letdown.

This is not intended to be an all-inclusive list. When a stable path of practices is being utilized with prudent self-pacing, any of these will generally be intermittent and short-lived as purification and opening advance within our nervous system, gradually giving way to a permanent condition of whole body ecstatic conductivity. Along with this will come an increased moral sensitivity – the feeling that what we are doing to others we are doing to ourselves, signifying a rising sense of *Oneness*, and leading to increasing harmonious and loving conduct.

It is possible that energy experiences like those listed above may not occur much at all, depending on the unique course of purification in our nervous system. Symptoms themselves are not prerequisites for progress. When we do have them, we will be wise to favor our practices and regard symptoms merely as *scenery*, or, if excessive, as feedback encouraging us to self-pace our practices and take additional remedial measures, as necessary. The objective is to maintain good progress with comfort and safety – not to have this or that experience overwhelming our practices and progress.

Experiences do not produce spiritual progress. Well-regulated practices over the long term do. It is essential to understand this important point.

This is the process of awakening kundalini. It is not an overnight event, as is commonly believed, no matter how dramatic any particular experience may be. The overall process of purification and opening can take many years, even with the best management of practices and their effects. It is a function of the unique matrix of obstructions that exists within each of us, and how long it takes to comfortably unwind it.

Due to the dramatic nature of some of the experiences that can occur, it is easy to underestimate the length and scope of the journey. One thing is for sure. If we are feeling that we have *arrived*, and are hankering to announce it to the world, it is a sign that we have not. The wisest course is to always favor the conduct of our practices over any experiences or flights of fancy that may arise, and just keep going.

Self-Pacing

If symptoms become excessive, it is a signal for us to self-pace (temporarily reduce) some or all of our practices. This does not mean running away from our yoga practices forever. It means moderating one or more of our practices to suit the conditions of our inner purification in the moment. Once the symptoms subside, we can slowly increase our practice again to find our best stable routine.

All of the symptoms listed above are the result of purification occurring in the nervous system. This is what we want, but not to the extreme. If we either accidentally or deliberately entertain the extremes of kundalini awakening, we may be driven away from yoga practices, which is falling off the path, even while being left in an ongoing difficult energy situation. Much better to keep things in a comfortable range and go for steady and safe purification and opening over the long term. So, we pace our progress by observing and adjusting the cause and effect in our practices. It is very do-able.

Some of our practices can help stabilize the symptoms of excess energy flow. This is especially true of spinal breathing pranayama. Many a case of kundalini difficulty has been aided by this wonderful practice, because it balances the ascending and descending energy currents in the spinal nerve and throughout the body. A set of easy and gentle asanas can help stabilize energy imbalances also, as can deep meditation. Each of us reacts differently to practices and we will find what works best for us in different circumstances over time.

Additional Remedies for Excess Kundalini Energy

Beyond what has been mentioned so far, there are other things we can do to help smooth our inner energies.

One of the best stabilizers of excess or unbalanced inner energy flows is daily exercise. This is why a yoga-friendly exercise program is included in the appendix. Exercise has a *grounding and integrating* effect on our inner energies. One of the best things we can do when the inner energies are acting up is take long walks. Very important.

Another method for quelling kundalini currents is a heavier diet for a time, and also moving the diet away from foods that are too acidic or stimulating. The ancient Indian health system of *Ayurveda* is especially good at offering diet guidelines and other means for reducing imbalances in the inner energies. This is discussed further in other AYP writings.

Finally, our lifestyle has an effect on our inner energies. Are we doing too much spiritual practice and not being out in the world enough? Are we working too much, or not enough? It is always important to favor a balance in our daily life, and especially when we are awakening our inner ecstatic energies. Do we keep enough of the right kind of company that is supportive of our spiritual commitment? Things like this can make a big difference in the stability of our inner energies in the formative stages, and hence in our spiritual progress.

The path of human spiritual transformation is not one-dimensional. It is multi-dimensional. This becomes experientially quite clear when our inner energies are awakening. We are becoming a pure channel of divine energy in the world. How we engage in the world will be influenced according to our own tendencies and choices. Ultimately, that means choosing the path of greatest ecstatic bliss. Kundalini has our highest expression and best interests inherent within it. The evolutionary force embedded within us will not falter in its purpose. We only need to adjust ourselves to accommodate it, and it will carry us ever higher.

Premature Kundalini Awakening

There has been the idea going around for a long time that the first step on the path to enlightenment is the awakening of kundalini. This is an incorrect understanding, or at least not one conducive to stable long term spiritual unfoldment. Relying first on kundalini to fuel our evolution is like relying on a building to hold itself up without a foundation under it. How realistic is that?

The result of such an approach is apparent in either case – a building teetering without its foundation, or kundalini running rampant in a person without a foundation or center. Both will be messy (or worse!) until the foundation has been put in place. It is much better to install the foundation *before* putting the building up, yes?

What is the foundation of kundalini? It is abiding *inner silence*, which is cultivated in daily deep meditation, and expanded into all aspects of life with samyama. Inner silence is also known as abiding *pure bliss consciousness*, the ground state and foundation of all manifest existence, including kundalini.

Daily practice of spinal breathing pranayama is also an important prerequisite to kundalini awakening. It stimulates and balances the rising and ascending energies in the spinal nerve. Spinal breathing can also be an effective remedy for out-of-balance kundalini energies.

So, the most important thing we can do as we approach the awakening of kundalini is begin our practices in the right place. If we begin prematurely with mudras and bandhas, particularly with breath retention added, we will be courting difficulty.

Crown practices can also create kundalini excesses and imbalances, especially if they are undertaken prior to prerequisite purification and opening provided by spinal breathing pranayama, deep meditation, and asanas, mudras and bandhas. This is why nearly all the practices in the AYP integrated system are oriented toward purification and opening of the spinal nerve (sushumna) from root to center brow, not root to crown (top of head). This is very important for sustaining long term stable growth with comfort and safety. Without comfort and safety, stable practice will go out the window, and steady growth will not be possible.

It is fine to be doing asanas as a stand-alone practice without taking up deep meditation first. Asanas are excellent for health and relaxation. However, ultimately, asanas will lead to more. There is little choice in the matter, because all of the limbs of yoga are interconnected through our nervous system.

As we become advanced in asanas, without incorporating deep meditation or spinal breathing, there can be the risk of an energy mishap. This is a common occurrence for long term asana practitioners. The kundalini energies eventually become aroused. When it happens, it is a call for deep meditation and spinal breathing, and possibly for the other remedial measures mentioned here.

Going from asanas straight to mudras and bandhas without deep meditation or spinal breathing in the picture can be like going out of the frying pan and into the fire. Mudras and bandhas are not primarily for quelling kundalini energies. They are for stimulating them. Mudras and bandhas can channel kundalini energy, but will usually not subdue it. Deep meditation and spinal breathing pranayama are, in part, for that, as well as the other means discussed above.

Kundalini awakening is a fact of life on the path of human spiritual transformation, no matter what system of practices or tradition we are following. It is much better to face kundalini and engage it in an intelligent and balanced process of unfoldment, rather than to try and avoid it and end up either with limited progress, or being thrown from pillar to post due to a lack of understanding and effective management. With good education and prudent application and pacing of a full range of yoga practices, we can enjoy the awakening of ecstatic kundalini and the many benefits of this great divine power and intelligence residing within us.

Mind-Boggling Energy and Intelligence

Beyond the challenges that an awakening kundalini may present, there are many positive and practical benefits. If we are measured in our practice, and effective in integrating the ecstatic energies within us, then we will find ourselves walking about with a great gift in our life, and with a rising spontaneous ability to bring blessings into the lives of others.

While we may seek our own enlightenment, we will only find it as we learn to give it away. That is how it works. The process of *giving* is an essential aspect of reaching the advanced stages of kundalini unfoldment and continuing progress on the path of yoga. The more we are able to give, the more we are able to receive in terms of our own spiritual evolution. The two processes are one and the same. This is not a moral guideline. Giving is simply part of the ongoing process of inner purification. There is no need to force it. Giving will happen in its own way as the divine energies continue to advance within us.

Giving what? That depends entirely on our personal inclinations. No one can define what the ideal path of another will be. It is within each of us, like a seed containing all that can be for us. All we must do is nurture that seed and allow it to grow to full maturity.

Yet, there is a commonality behind every seed. It is the reality of inner silence and ecstatic conductivity (kundalini), and the blending of these in action. This is how divine energy flows through us into the world.

From the ecstatic kundalini side, there are tell-tale characteristics. The energy within us increases in flow as purification advances within our nervous system. As inner obstacles dissolve, kundalini manifests with increasing power. What we find is mind-boggling energy and intelligence flowing through us. Whether we claim this as our own or not is a matter of how we see ourselves. We may see the flow as an expression of our own being, or we may see ourselves as a channel of the flow coming from the divine within. Either way, it happens, and we find ourselves able to do what before might have seemed impossible.

The energy of kundalini is physical, psychological and emotional. It is as though we have tapped into a magical source of nutrition beyond food alone. In fact, part of the neurobiology of kundalini occurs in the digestive system, where food, sexual essences and air are combined to produce a luminous mint-like substance called *soma* that energizes every cell and nerve in our body.

Most remarkable is that the energy of kundalini is intelligent beyond human reckoning. The insights and revelations are such that we can only surrender to what is being revealed to us from within. All that we think and do becomes colored by a great river of love. We are obliged to utilize the surging energy and intelligence within the context of the river of love that delivers these qualities from within us. So, whether we regard this flow to be our own self or to be a divine deliverance coming through us, it will contain seemingly unbounded energy, intelligence, love, and all that naturally spins off from these divine qualities in our daily activity.

By the time we reach the advanced stages of kundalini awakening, our nervous system has evolved from a 100-watt light bulb to become a 1000-watt light bulb. And it will shine brightly...

Enlightenment – Outpouring Divine Love

The definitions of enlightenment vary greatly. Every knowledge system seems to have its own description. Ultimately, enlightenment, if there is such a thing, can only be determined by direct experience.

Is enlightenment divine illumination in the physical sense of energy (light) radiating from us? Is it manifested as profound wisdom? Is enlightenment love? All of these have been mentioned in the classical definitions, and perhaps all of these are aspects of the thing we call enlightenment. These also happen to be the known qualities of an advancing kundalini awakening.

Three Steps of Enlightenment

Looking at enlightenment from another point of view, we can see a three-step process at work, leading to the same result we have been discussing above.

If we begin with deep meditation, we are immediately laying the foundation of the entire spiritual journey – inner silence (pure bliss consciousness). If we track the rise of inner silence, what we find is a gradual expansion and stabilization of it, giving rise to the experience of an inner *silent witness*, present at all times during daily activity, dreaming sleep, and deep dreamless sleep. This ongoing presence of the witness can be described as the first step of enlightenment. We also call it the first enlightenment milestone. It is freedom from the ups and downs of life.

But there is more.

Sometime after beginning deep meditation, we can begin spinal breathing pranayama, and later on be adding mudras and bandhas, one-by-one, according to the principles of self-pacing. We may have added asanas in front of our sitting routine early on, or perhaps we were doing asanas before we began sitting practices – either way is fine.

With the systematic addition of these breathing and physical techniques over time, we will at some point feel the rise of ecstatic conductivity occurring. Along with this comes a gradually clearing perception of our inner ecstatic energies – it has been called inner seeing. Profound beauty is experienced in this stage, and the subsequent effects in the heart (a melting) invariably lead to a devotional relationship with the ecstatic energies. It can be within the culture and religious tradition we have been brought up in, or it can be completely individualized. It is a choice we make along the path. However it may occur, the underlying experience is of ecstatic conductivity (kundalini) coming up throughout the body, and also seen and felt in the external environment. This is the second step of enlightenment, also called the second milestone.

As inner silence and ecstatic conductivity are coming up simultaneously in the body, they mingle and merge over time to become a new, combined experience. It is ecstasy moving in stillness and stillness moving in ecstasy. We also call it *stillness in action*. Whatever we call it, there is a new dynamic that involves both of these inner qualities – inner silence and ecstatic conductivity.

When stillness becomes mobile on the waves of ecstatic energy coursing through us and out into our activity, we again find the qualities of an awakening kundalini – vast flows of energy, intelligence and love, with all of this pouring out from a permanent, unshakable sea of silence within us. It is the unity of inner and outer life, the fruition of yoga. This is the third step in the enlightenment process, the third milestone.

In reality, we may experience varying degrees of the three steps of enlightenment at any time along the way on our journey. It is helpful to recognize them, and their relationship to the practices we are doing, for inspiration and for use in self-pacing as necessary.

Remember, we are managing cause and effect in our practice routine, not just blindly doing practices and hoping for the best. We would not drive a car that way, would we? And neither should we open the divine doorway of our nervous system that way. If we do, we will be in for a rough ride, and probably not arrive in a timely fashion. With good understanding of the methods and dynamics of practice, we will have a much quicker and smoother ride.

Asanas, mudras and bandhas have an important role to play on the ecstatic side of the enlightenment equation. If undertaken and managed as part of a fully integrated program of practices, these physical techniques can make a huge difference in our spiritual progress, speeding us along comfortably and safely with the awakening of ecstatic kundalini.

It is up to each of us to decide when and how we will conduct our spiritual journey. No one can make these decisions for us. There is great wisdom within us, encouraging and guiding us every step of our journey. If we listen, we will know the way.

With good tools and prudent practice, we cannot miss. That is because we already contain within us everything that is needed to live our life in the fullness of unshakable inner silence, ecstatic bliss, and outpouring divine love.

It is our destiny.

Appendix

A Yoga-Friendly Exercise Program

There are many definitions of fitness. As they say, "Beauty is in the eye of the beholder."

For purposes of spiritual practice, fitness means keeping the body in good tone and flexible externally and internally, which can be done with daily walking or other light aerobic-style exercise, light calisthenics and isometrics for all muscle groups, and, of course, yoga asanas. Something like Tai Chi is also good, which builds a good connection between the physical and spiritual dimensions of us in a grounding way.

For the body builder (or any physically oriented athlete) that is not enough. He or she will want to do much more with the muscles. The practices must be aimed at the goal.

For spiritual practice, the things mentioned above are enough. For other definitions of fitness it will be something else.

There is no rule that says a body builder or any other kind of athlete cannot become a yogi or yogini. There is nothing that says one can't do both if so inclined. It is just a question of what one's interests are. Here we believe in free choice and in each person taking personal responsibility for their life.

Light aerobic exercise for the cardiovascular system, as well as some calisthenics and isometrics for toning all the muscle groups, are good to help maintain the body in suitable condition for yoga practices. When these are done in addition to daily asana practice, then a good blend of strength and limberness can be achieved. For those who do not have an exercise program, some suggestions are included here. Even if you do have an exercise program, maybe a few of these suggestions will be helpful.

Aerobic Exercise

So, what comes first in exercise? Cardiovascular conditioning is fundamental to good health, so let's start with aerobic exercise. What is aerobic exercise? It is activity that causes the body to process more oxygen. Doing such activity on a regular basis strengthens the cardiovascular system (heart and blood circulation). Aerobic exercise is engaging in activity that causes the heart rate to go up for a period of time. Somewhere between 10 and 30 minutes of elevated heart rate is considered to be a good aerobic exercise session. With this, the lungs, the heart and the circulatory system will be moving more oxygen to the muscles, tissues and organs. That is what "aerobic" means – processing oxygen. The more conditioned our cardiovascular system is, the better we feel, and the better we are for yoga too.

What are some good aerobic exercises? Walking is an effective way to get aerobic exercise. Not only does it give the cardiovascular system a workout; it also grounds the inner energies. That is why taking long walks is recommended to help stabilize kundalini imbalances. Other aerobic exercises are jogging, biking, swimming, stair climbing, rowing, lively dancing, or anything that requires constant physical movement producing an elevated heart rate (not too much) for at least 10 minutes.

As with a yoga routine, an exercise program is only good to the extent that we can maintain regular practice. Taking a long walk once a week will do some good, but it will not condition our cardiovascular system significantly. If we want the benefits of conditioning, exercise at least every other day is very important. Daily is even better.

Once we get started with an exercise program, the trick is to keep going, keeping to a schedule of daily (or every other day) aerobic exercise for a set time and/or distance. The goal is to get our heart rate up 20-40 beats per minute above normal and keep it there for the time of our exercise.

Make sure you don't have any health limitations before undertaking an aerobic exercise program. If in doubt, check with your doctor first.

Muscle Toning

Whatever aerobic exercise we are doing, we will get some muscle toning out of it. But the chances are it will be limited to our legs or arms, depending on the type of aerobic exercise we are doing. The main benefit from aerobic exercise is cardiovascular conditioning, which is what we want. What about the rest of our body – all those hundreds of muscles that enable us to function in daily life? Having them in good shape is an important support to yoga as well.

We live in the age of the "gym." Everyone goes to the gym. Well, almost everyone. But do we really have to go that far to get a good muscle toning all over our body? And do we really need all that equipment? When we don't have a gym in our house, and don't have time to go to one, what can we do to keep in shape? It is possible to keep all of our major muscle groups in good tone without exercise equipment, and without even going out of our house. The way to do this is with a concentrated routine of light calisthenics and isometric exercises. You will be amazed to see how much can be done in only a few minutes.

Let's talk about a streamlined routine of light calisthenics and isometrics that can be done at home in 5-10 minutes covering all the muscle groups. If you do these every day (every other day, at least), you will feel dramatically stronger within a few weeks, With this exercise routine, your muscles will become firm and toned, without the huge bulging physique. Before all the fitness machines came along, methods such as these were used to build large muscles too, and still can be.

So here is a streamlined muscle toning routine for you to try:

1. **Easy Push-ups** – Everyone hates push-ups, present company included. But there is a way to do them without the pain and anguish, or like feeling like you just joined the football team or the military. They are very good for the chest, arms and back muscles. Here is the trick. Get two chairs, or anything about chair height, and hold yourself up with your hands on those in push-up position. Not too bad? Now come down a little, not too far, and back up. That's one. Now do 25 of those, coming down just enough to put a little tension on your arms and chest muscles. Only come down far enough so you know you can finish the 25 repetitions, even if it is only dipping an inch or two. If you are in good shape you can come down further, and do the 25 repetitions that way. In other words, this is *self-paced*. Once you get comfortable doing 25 repetitions, maybe in a couple of weeks, raise the repetitions up to 50. Maybe you will not be going deep on each push-

up, but you will be doing 50. Then you can work with that over time, and see how it goes, never putting yourself in the position of over-exerting. Just an easy 50, that's all. You will be amazed what that will do in a few weeks, and you will never have to strain like you are in army boot camp.

2. **Isometric Curls** – Stand up with feet about shoulder-width apart. Place the heel of your left hand on the heel of your right hand. Now lift your right hand up toward your chest with a curling motion, resisting firmly with your left hand as you go, and then all the way back down. Do 50 of these curls, resisting enough so you will get a good muscle toning, but not so much that you can't make it to 50 repetitions. Now do the same thing on the other side. This is a dynamic isometric for toning the arm and shoulder muscles.

3. **Easy Knee Bends** – Still standing with feet about shoulder-width, clasp your hands behind your head. Do a small knee bend, and another, and another, all the way up to 50. Don't go to too deep – just deep enough so you can make it to 50 without overdoing it. If your legs are in good shape go a little deeper. Self-pacing. This gives the upper legs a good toning. If time is short (as it often is), you can do the knee bends at the same time as the isometric curls. If you do knee bends with curls (one bend for each curl) all the way through while doing both arms, that will be 100 knee bends. You can stop the knee bends at 50, or go for the whole 100. You are standing there

anyway, right? If you don't go too deep with the knee bends, 100 should not be a problem. Self-pacing. It is up to you.

4. **Neck Toning** – Now we will work on the neck muscles in four directions. First, place the fingers of both hands on your forehead and push your head forward and down against firm resistance from your hands 20 times. Now, place your fingers on the back of your head and push your head back and down against firm resistance from your hands 20 times. With the heel of your right hand against the right side of your head above the ear, push your head to the right and down 20 times against firm resistance. Then, on the left side, do the same thing. With these four isometrics, you will gain a lot of neck toning and strength.

5. **Foot and Calf Toning** – Take one of those chairs and put it against the wall. Step up onto the edge of it, with your heels hanging over the edge. Place a hand on the wall for balance. Now, lower your heels and lift them back up as high as you comfortably can, standing on your toes on the edge of the chair. This can also be done on the bottom step of a flight of stairs. Do 50 repetitions of this, using the same method of self-pacing so as not to overdo it. The key is to do 50. This is very good for toning the foot, ankle and calf muscles.

6. **Easy Sit-ups** – Lie on your back on the bed or other soft surface. Anchoring your feet in some way is suggested. Sit up and clasp your hands

behind your head. Now go back down about half way, and sit up and lean forward toward your knees. Each time you come up, twist your torso so one elbow goes toward the opposite knee. Reverse the twist coming up each time. Do that to 30 repetitions. These are sit-ups, only we are regulating the amount of tension placed on the abdomen in a way so anyone can do these. Only go back down far enough so you can easily do the sit-ups for the 30 repetitions. The toning is mainly in the upper abdominal muscles. Those with abdominal muscles not in good shape can just lean back a little to do easy sit-ups. Those with strong abdominal muscles can go all the way down, as long as the 30 repetitions can be completed. It should be easy for everyone, with good upper abdominal muscle toning occurring, no matter what level one is working at.

7. **Easy Leg Lifts** – Now lie on your back, anchor your hands over your head and lift your legs straight up, keeping the knees fairly straight. Let the legs go down toward the bed, and then back up straight in the air. Do 30 of these leg lifts, keeping in mind that you should only go down as far with your legs as you can comfortably lift them back up for 30 repetitions. Self-pacing. This tones the lower abdominal muscles.

That is just seven exercises. They can all be done in 5-10 minutes. Don't be fooled by the simplicity of these. This is a sophisticated, streamlined routine of exercises that will tone all the muscles in the body. It took years to refine it down to this level of efficiency. As with all the practices we discuss in AYP, these exercises are optimized for simplicity and power. The effective use of self-pacing allows anyone in any condition to begin toning the muscles.

For those who are in excellent physical shape, the exercises can be taken much further than the minimums, including increasing the repetitions, as comfortable.

Exercise, both aerobic and muscle toning, should not be done right before yoga practices. Doing them right after sitting practices and rest is good, or at any other time during the day. If you do the exercises at least every other day, you will find great benefits for both the short term and the long term.

Further Reading and Support

Yogani is an American spiritual scientist who, for more than thirty years, has been integrating ancient techniques from around the world which cultivate human spiritual transformation. The approach he has developed is non-sectarian, and open to all. In the order published, his books include:

Advanced Yoga Practices – Easy Lessons for Ecstatic Living
A large user-friendly textbook providing 240 detailed lessons on the AYP integrated system of yoga practices.

The Secrets of Wilder – A Novel
The story of young Americans discovering and utilizing actual secret practices leading to human spiritual transformation.

The AYP Enlightenment Series
Easy-to-read instruction books on yoga practices, including:

- *Deep Meditation – Pathway to Personal Freedom*
- *Spinal Breathing Pranayama – Journey to Inner Space*
- *Tantra – Discovering the Power of Pre-Orgasmic Sex*
- *Asanas, Mudras and Bandhas – Awakening Ecstatic Kundalini*
- *Samyama – Cultivating Stillness in Action* (2nd half 2006)
- *Diet, Shatkarmas and Amaroli – Yogic Nutrition and Cleansing for Health and Spirit* (1st half 2007)
- *Self Inquiry – Dawn of the Witness and the End of Suffering* (1st half 2007)
- *Bhakti and Karma Yoga – The Science of Devotion and Liberation Through Action* (2nd half 2007)
- *Eight Limbs of Yoga – The Structure and Pacing of Self-Directed Spiritual Practice* (2nd half 2007)

For up-to-date information on the writings of Yogani, and for the free *AYP Support Forums*, please visit:

www.advancedyogapractices.com

Printed in the United States
89815LV00001BA/23/A